Random Walk and Diffusion Models

Wolf Schwarz

Random Walk and Diffusion Models

An Introduction for Life and Behavioral Scientists

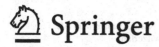 Springer

Wolf Schwarz
Research Methods in Human Sciences
University of Potsdam
Potsdam, Brandenburg, Germany

ISBN 978-3-031-12102-9 ISBN 978-3-031-12100-5 (eBook)
https://doi.org/10.1007/978-3-031-12100-5

Mathematics Subject Classification: 60J70, 92D50, 91E10

This Springer imprint is published by the registered company Springer Nature Switzerland AG
The registered company address is: Gewerbestrasse 11, 6330 Cham, Switzerland

We often felt that there is not less, and perhaps even more, beauty in the result of analysis than there is to be found in mere contemplation.

Niko Tinbergen, *Curious Naturalists* (1958).

Preface

In recent decades, random walk and diffusion models have become quite popular in areas far beyond their traditional background in physics. Those areas include biology, both at a neuronal and a behavioral level, population genetics, ecology, sociology, sports science, public health applications, and models of perception, cognition, and decision-making, to name just a few typical examples. This is in my view an exciting and encouraging development, as it can help to bridge the gap between experimental, or empirical, and theoretical branches in the several fields mentioned.

One serious problem in this context, which I noted frequently in lecturing on random walk and diffusion models, is that master's or even PhD students in the life sciences typically have a background in mathematical and quantitative modeling that is quite different from what standard accounts of these models assume or require. These accounts cover the material in a dense, compact style when for life science students detailed, careful, and more intuitive step-by-step explanations would be most helpful. Furthermore, the general orientation of most standard references, as exemplified by their selection of applied examples –if there are any at all– often does not connect well to the context and the conceptual background that is typical of applications in the life and behavioral sciences.

The present book seeks to remedy this mismatch, primarily by

- Aiming at the most accessible explanation of the formal concepts
- Limiting the content covered to basic standard models
- Providing detailed and intuitive step-by-step explanations
- Moving smoothly from the simplest to more complex models
- Accessing and explaining the same basic results from different conceptual approaches
- Referring to applied examples in the literature, beyond the more traditional natural science background
- Providing a separate chapter illustrating successful and original applications of random walk and diffusion models in the life and behavioral sciences

- Giving explicit references to early landmark contributions which often provide the beginning student with crystal-clear expositions of basic conceptual ideas
- Providing a set of well-chosen, informative, and deepening exercises

Despite this general orientation, the present Introduction is clearly not a "Diffusion made easy" book, trading substance for comfort. It is true that many central ideas related to random walk and diffusion models are intrinsically elegant, having a beautiful, elementary structure. This said, the conceptual representation and the formal techniques required to describe, to analyze, and to apply these models are neither trivial nor familiar in the life and behavioral sciences. The present Introduction does not aim to conceal this fact; it guides the reader carefully through the details of conceptual notions and formal techniques required to formulate and analyze random walk and diffusion models. Its aim would be fulfilled if after studying it, say, a biologist or a sports scientist would be fit to turn with confidence to established standard references, several of which are listed in the References.

My approach in this book is often heuristic, and I stress the conceptual interpretation of the formalisms. The main aim is to present random walk and diffusion models at the conceptual and technical level at which they are actually applied in the life and behavioral sciences. The only mathematical prerequisites are to be familiar with the main notions of calculus, and to have some previous exposure to the basic concepts of probability theory, a level corresponding, for example, to the masterful treatment of Stewart (2012), or to Stewart and Day (2016). Slightly more advanced technical tools such as partial derivatives or moment-generating functions are explained and used in a clearly heuristic, engineer–like manner. The exercises at the end of the chapters serve to complement and deepen the main treatment of the topics. They help, at different levels of difficulty, to gain practice with the approaches and techniques, and they play an important role in the active acquisition and mastery of the required skills.

Potsdam, Germany   Wolf Schwarz

Contents

Chapter 1
Introduction

1.1 Random Walk and Diffusion Models in the Life and the Behavioral Sciences

In 1827, the Scottish botanist Robert Brown examined under a microscope grains of pollen of a wildflower plant suspended in water. He noted that the pollen burst at their corners and emitted minute particles which jiggled around in the water in a random, jittery fashion, a phenomenon now known as Brownian motion.

The motion process first observed by Brown represents a prototype of a scenario in which a quantity of interest moves in an at least partly unpredictable fashion across time, although superimposed systematic trends or drifts may be present as well. Randomly evolving processes of this type are often described in terms of quantitative concepts technically known as random walk and diffusion models. These concepts form the main topic of the present book and are explained in detail in later chapters. To a large degree, random walk and diffusion models were originally developed in physics where they are used to explain, for example, how the mean displacement of small particles per time unit depends on temperature, on the radius of the particle, and on the viscosity of the suspension. Eminent physicists such as Albert Einstein, Marian von Smoluchowski, Paul Langevin, or Erwin Schrödinger formulated these models and investigated their basic properties, which testifies to the importance attached to the conceptual notions on which they were built.

Inspired by these developments, other researchers sought to apply these quantitative concepts to the sort of spatial movement processes of more interest, for example, to biologists. As shown in Fig. 1.1, Przibram (1913) recorded the two-dimensional trajectory of paramecia (oblong unicellular organisms whose length is about 0.1 mm); he confirmed that their irregular movement corresponds to basic predictions derived from random walk and diffusion models. Since the original study of Przibram (1913), there is a strong tradition in biology and ecology which seeks to investigate and explain the ways in which animals move around in terms of

© Springer Nature Switzerland AG 2022
W. Schwarz, *Random Walk and Diffusion Models*,
https://doi.org/10.1007/978-3-031-12100-5_1

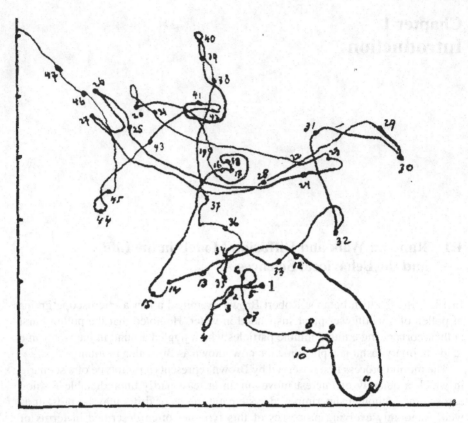

Fig. 1.1 Drawing from Przibram (1913), the earliest application of random walk and diffusion models to the movement of animals. The hand-drawn line represents the trajectory of a paramecium, a unicellular ciliate. The numbers next to the line indicate the successive positions of the animal every 4 s, as signaled by a metronome. Aided by a microscope, Przibram used a mechanical tracking device which he operated while he was observing the animal. One unit of the axes corresponds to 0.27 mm on the slide of the microscope; the typical length of a paramecium is about 0.10 mm

the basic notions inherent to these models; some typical related studies are described in Sect. 7.4.

In many applications of random walk and diffusion models, the real physical space in which Brown's pollen grains and Przibram's paramecia moved around is replaced by a more metaphorical, conceptual state space. For example, the way in which prices of common stocks at exchange markets vary over time is often described using random walk and diffusion models. In this particular application, the "movements" are the price changes, and the uni-dimensional state space of the model refers to the range of possible stock prices (for a non-technical early exposition, see Fama 1965). Similarly, the temporal evolution of the home team lead in basketball matches can be interpreted as a diffusion process (Schwarz 2012; Stern 1994). As shown in Fig. 1.2, the state (i.e., the home team lead) of this process

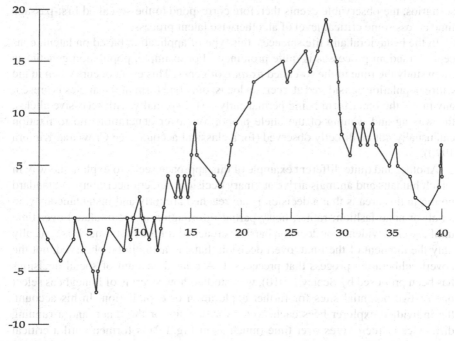

Fig. 1.2 The home team lead (ordinate) is the score difference of the home minus the away team, considered as a function of time (abscissa; in minutes) into the match. The example shown refers to basketball; negative values to the left of the graph indicate that the away team led during much of the first 10 min. Then the home team caught up, reached a maximum lead of 19 points after 28 min, and eventually closely won the match with a score difference of 4. For details, see Sect. 7.5 and Schwarz (2012)

at any time is the running difference of points scored by the home team minus the points scored by the away team.

Even though the state space in these examples is conceptual rather than physical, it is still true that the actual movements (the price or score changes) can be directly observed in an essentially continuous manner. Many important applications of random walk and diffusion models in the behavioral and life sciences address situations in which the hypothesized underlying random process is not directly observable but only certain functionals defined on it are. For example, Whitmore (1979) modelled the length of employment after which staff members quit their job in organizations. He assumed that there exists a *latent* variable that may be conceptualized as job attachment and whose level fluctuates over time. When this variable reaches for the first time a critical level (the separation threshold), then the employee will quit the job. With this type of application, only a single point in time is directly observable, namely, the moment at which notice is given. In these scenarios, the observable events therefore correspond to the so-called first-passage time across some critical level of an otherwise latent process.

In the behavioral and life sciences, this type of application based on latent, conceptual random processes is quite prominent. For example, population geneticists often study the time to the so-called *fixation* of genes. This event occurs when in the entire population considered at a certain locus, only one form of the alleles is present any more, the other form being permanently lost. Especially with recessive alleles, the waxing and waning of the allele proportions over generations up to fixation can usually not be directly observed (for a classical account, see Crow and Kimura 1970).

Another and quite different example of this approach seeks to explain the way in which humans and animals arrive at binary decisions under uncertainty. A standard notion in this area is that a decision is not reached abruptly and instantaneously, in an all-or-none fashion; rather, noisy partial information is accumulated over time until a preset evidence or decision barrier is reached for the first time. It is typically only the moment of the final, overt decision that can actually be observed, not the covert deliberating process that precedes it. A related account of social decisions has been proposed by Seeley (2010), who studied how swarms of honeybees select one of two potential sites for further exploration or exploitation. In his account, the individual explorer bees each "vote" for one site or the other, and a running difference of their votes over time (much as in Fig. 1.2) is formed until a critical upper or lower threshold is reached for the first time. Seeley coined the concise term "bee democracy" for this process of collective decision-making.

In Chap. 7, we will review several further characteristic applications of random walk and diffusion models in different areas of the behavioral and life sciences.

Since the earliest applications reviewed above, the study and analysis of random walk and diffusion models has become a highly developed and specialized branch of the quantitative sciences that often appears in an austere technical guise. Formal abstraction is, to be sure, a necessary requirement for any deeper understanding of random processes. However, it also tends to cloud the intrinsic simplicity and elegance of the subject—in particular, the versatility and plausibility of the basic mechanisms generating random walks and diffusion processes. We present and discuss two important historic examples, Galton's board and Fick's laws, which illustrate these core generating mechanisms in an elementary and lucid manner. At the same time, we will use these examples to introduce some important basic concepts and notions. The first example, Galton's board, refers to discrete spatial steps executed at regular time steps. The second example, Fick's laws, treats space and time as essentially continuous quantities. However, conceptually both examples rest on very similar elementary ideas.

1.2 Two Historic Examples

1.2.1 Galton's Board

With the deeper understanding of thermodynamics and electromagnetism, and the attendant rise of steam engines and electric generators, nineteenth-century science developed a marked tendency to represent conceptual ideas in terms of mechanical notions and to embody such ideas in the form of mechanical devices.

Galton's board is a typical example of this mechanical era. It embodies basic probabilistic notions as a simple physical device that illustrates how binomial distributions, and thus the most elementary diffusion processes, arise.

As indicated in Fig. 1.3, it consists of an upright board with interleaved rows of wedges. Balls enter from a narrow funnel at the top and bounce with equal probability either to the left or to the right as they hit the wedges on their way downward. Eventually, they are collected into bins at the bottom.

In Fig. 1.3, the vertical dimension corresponds to the number of steps made, that is, to time, assuming a constant ball speed. The horizontal dimension corresponds to the spatial displacement, labeled 0, 1, 2, 3, and 4 from left to right, meaning that

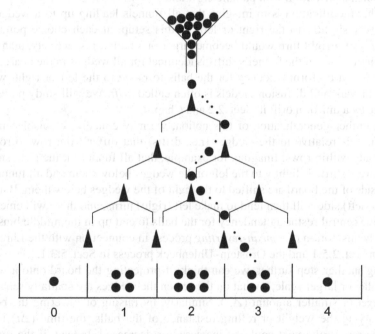

Fig. 1.3 Balls enter Galton's board from a funnel at the top and bounce with equal probability either left or right as they hit the wedges in successive rows. Eventually, they are collected into bins at the bottom. The board shown has four rows and illustrates the dotted path of one ball that falls three times to the right and one time to the left, ending up in the bin labeled 3. The number of balls in the bins illustrates the relative frequencies with which balls will end up in the various bins

in the example of Fig. 1.3, the ball enters the board at position 2 and that each step from one row to the next has a size of $\pm\frac{1}{2}$ of one bin width. Thus, the frequencies indicated in the five bins at the bottom refer to the probability that the ball has moved to position $x = 0, \ldots, 4$ after four steps. The essential insight is that in order for the ball to end up at position x, it must, in some arbitrary order, turn x times to the right and thus $4 - x$ times to the left. There are $\binom{4}{x}$ ways to select those x right turns from among the four turns in all, corresponding to so many different paths ending up at position x. Each individual path has a probability equal to $\left(\frac{1}{2}\right)^4$, but there are more paths that end up in the middle bins. For example, there is only one path—turning to the right at every wedge—that ends up at $x = 4$. This path is no less likely than any other, but it is the only way to end up in the rightmost bin, which explains why so few balls finish in that bin.

This basic scheme may be generalized in several important ways that we will address in later chapters of this book. A natural generalization is to think of a board with an arbitrary number n of rows. If on its way to the bins at the bottom a ball makes x right turns and $n - x$ left turns, it will end up at a position with a net displacement to the right equal to $[x - (n - x)]/2 = x - n/2$, relative to its start position. The probability of this final position is equal to $\binom{n}{x}\left(\frac{1}{2}\right)^n$, obtained from the binomial distribution with parameters n and $p = \frac{1}{2}$.

Another modification is to imagine that all funnels leading up to a wedge are shifted very slightly to the right or left. In this setup, at each choice point, the probability of a right turn would become larger or smaller, respectively, than one-half. If the amount of the funnel's shifts is identical for all wedges in the board, then there will be a uniform tendency for the balls to move to the left or right, which in random walk and diffusion models is often called *drift*. We will study processes governed by a uniform drift in Sect. 2.2 and Chap. 4.

As a further generalization of this notion, we may conceive of displacements of the funnels relative to the wedges (i.e., drifts) that differ from row to row or horizontally within rows. Imagine, for example, that all funnels at the right side of the board are shifted slightly to the left of the wedges below them and all funnels at the left side of the board are shifted to the right of the wedges below them. Balls on the right (left) side will then tend to make left (right) turns, and there will emerge a systematic central restoring tendency for the balls to end up in the middle bins. We will study this notion of a *mean-reverting* process in connection with the Ehrenfest model in Sect. 2.5.1 and the Ornstein–Uhlenbeck process in Sect. 5.3.1.

Going another step further, we can think of projecting the board onto a screen in a smaller or larger scale, so that on the screen the wedges are spatially separated by a larger or smaller amount (Δx). Similarly, by raising or lowering the board, or by varying the weight or rolling resistance of the balls, the time (Δt) to get from one row to the next could be increased or decreased. Indeed, if the row-to-row speed is very high, and the wedge separations are very small, the path of any ball would appear to an observer more and more as a smooth, continuous movement in space and time. Thus, in a final step, we can appeal to the central limit theorem

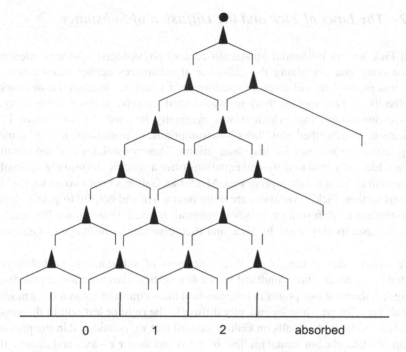

0   1   2   absorbed

Fig. 1.4 The setup is similar to Fig. 1.3, but when the ball exceeds a horizontal displacement that corresponds to the separation between bin 2 and bin 3, then it drops permanently into the bottom bin labeled "absorbed"

of probability theory (Ross 2019), according to which for large n, the position x at time $t = n \, \Delta t$ represents the result of a large number of independent, additive steps and thus tends (for fixed t) to a normal distribution in the spatial coordinate. We will describe this sort of limiting process in more detail in Chaps. 3 and 4.

A somewhat different modification of Galton's binomial scheme, illustrated in Fig. 1.4, is to restrict the free evolution of the balls as they run through the board. We may attach to each row at the distance of (say) a to the right of the starting position an absorbing bin so that the ball will stop its downward course in this bin when it first reaches the position a. Running a large number of balls through the modified board in Fig. 1.4 with an absorbing bin at a, we can study if and when balls first reach a position at a distance a from the start. This is the simplest form of including an *absorbing state* which once reached is never left again. The probability that this state is ever reached and the corresponding first-passage time distribution associated with reaching that state will be recurring topics in all later chapters.

1.2.2   The Laws of Fick and the Diffusion of Substance

Adolf Fick was an influential nineteenth-century physiologist who was interested
in measuring and explaining the diffusion of substances across membranes. To
study this process, he did careful experiments in which he measured how quickly
salt dissolves (i.e., spreads out) in water-filled vessels, starting from a small
cross-section (layer) into which it was originally injected. In his classic 1855
publication, he described two "laws"—assumptions, or postulates, might be more
fitting terms—to account for his observations. These postulates and the detailed
way in which they lead to diffusion equations offer a specific, intuitively accessible
approach to account for such processes. Much like Galton's board considered in the
previous section, Fick's postulates are quite instructive and helpful to gain a clearer
understanding of diffusion processes in general. In the following, we first explain
the basic assumptions made by Fick and then consider some ways to generalize
them.

We assume that at time $t = 0$, a unit mass of substance (=probability) is
injected into a horizontal cylindrical vessel at a vertical cross-section at coordinate
x_0. Fig. 1.5 shows at two points in time this unit mass equivalently as a large number
of small particles which independently diffuse to the right or left within the vessel,
much like the individual balls on Galton's board that we considered in the previous
section. We take the horizontal midline of the vessel as our $x-$axis and assume that
the vessel extends to the left and right of x_0 with infinite length. For the moment, we
also ignore the fact that the particles are confined (i.e., reflected) by the cylindrical
vessel.

Denote the amount of mass (or the proportion of particles) which at time t is to
the left of x by $F(x, t)$, and denote the associated concentration by $f(t, x) = \frac{\partial F}{\partial x}$. In
probabilistic terms, F corresponds to a distribution function, and f to the associated
density at time t. For example, we must have for any t that $F(-\infty, t) = 0$ and
$F(+\infty, t) = 1$; also, F is nondecreasing in x. On the other hand, if we focus
on a given, fixed value of x, then $F(x, t)$ may be an increasing, a decreasing, or
even a constant function of t. Note the asymmetric roles played by x and t: $f(x, t)$
integrates for any t across all x to unity, but this statement is not correct for a given,
fixed value of x across all t.

The laws of Fick relate changes of concentration f in time and space. Their basic
statement is this: the amount of substance passing in a short time interval $[t, t + \Delta t]$
from left to right through a cross-section of the vessel at x is proportional to:

 (i) the length, Δt, of the (short) time interval
 (ii) the gradient (the slope or derivative) of the concentration f at x at time t.

The constant of proportionality is negative and is denoted by $-D$, where $D >$
0. Summarizing these two postulates formally, Fick assumed that the amount of
substance passing through x in $[t, t + \Delta t]$ is equal to $-D \frac{\partial f}{\partial x} \Delta t$.

Some comments will help to motivate the nature of Fick's assumptions. First,
"the amount" is meant as a net flow from left to right, and this net flow may be

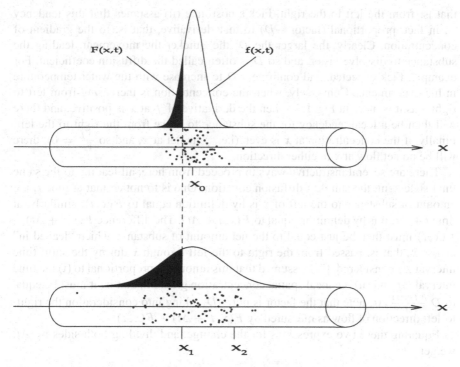

Fig. 1.5 At time $t = 0$, a unit mass of substance (shown here as many particles) is injected into a horizontal cylindrical vessel at a vertical cross-section at coordinate x_0. Taking the horizontal midline of the vessel as the x−axis, the local concentration (density) at x at time t is denoted as $f(x, t)$. The proportion of mass (particles) below (to the left of) x at time t is denoted as $F(x, t) = \int_{-\infty}^{x} f(u, t) du$. The top panel shows the concentration at time t and the bottom panel at a later time $t' > t$

positive, zero, or negative. For example, a negative flow would mean that at x (more) substance flows from the right to the left. As is discussed below, we might think of this as the net result of a left-to-right stream of particles minus a right-to-left stream of particles, but for now, it may be easier to think of it in terms of the resulting net flow.

Second, assumption (i) simply states that for short time intervals Δt, we expect nearly additive relations. For example, the amount of substance passing x in two short, successive time intervals would be expected to be about twice the amount passing in each of these short time intervals individually. This means that the (small) flow in the first interval will not fundamentally change the flow during the second interval.

Finally, the central substantive assumption is part (ii). Note that when (going from left to right) the concentration f is decreasing—as it is at x_2 in Fig. 1.5—then the derivative of f at x is negative. According to (ii), there will then be a local tendency for the substance to move from higher to lower levels of concentration, that is, from the left to the right. Fick's postulate (ii) assumes that this tendency is, in fact, proportional (factor $-D$) to that derivative, that is, to the gradient of concentration. Clearly, the larger the D, the quicker the movement, leading the substance to dissolve faster, and so D is often called the diffusion coefficient. For example, Fick expected, and confirmed, D to increase with the water temperature in his experiments. Conversely, when the concentration is increasing from left to right—as it is at x_1 in Fig. 1.5—then the derivative of f at x is positive, and there will then be a local tendency for the substance to move from the right to the left. Finally, if the concentration at x is even (i.e., f is flat at x, and so $\frac{\partial f}{\partial x} = 0$), there will be no net flow at x in either direction.

There are several instructive ways to proceed from here, all leading to the same final statement, the simplest diffusion equation. One is to notice that at time t, the amount of substance to the left of x is by definition equal to $F(x, t)$; similarly, at time $t + \Delta t$, it is by definition equal to $F(x, t + \Delta t)$. The difference $F(x, t + \Delta t) - F(x, t)$ must then be just equal to the net amount of substance which "leaked in" across x, that is, passed from the right to the left through x during the short time interval Δt considered. Fick assumed that this amount is proportional to (i) the time interval Δt and (ii) the local spatial concentration gradient; that is, it must be equal to $D \frac{\partial f(x,t)}{\partial x} \Delta t$; note that the factor is not $-D$, taking into consideration the right-to-left direction of flow as measured by $F(x, t + \Delta t) - F(x, t)$.

Equating these two expressions for the change, and dividing both sides by Δt, we get

$$\frac{F(x, t + \Delta t) - F(x, t)}{\Delta t} = D \frac{\partial f}{\partial x} \tag{1.1}$$

According to the definition of a derivative (Stewart 2012, ch. 2, and Sect. 3.2.1), for $\Delta t \to 0$, this gives

$$\frac{\partial F}{\partial t} = D \frac{\partial f}{\partial x} \tag{1.2}$$

Also, as explained above, the concentration $f(t, x) = \frac{\partial F}{\partial x}$; therefore, if we differentiate both sides of Eq. (1.2) with respect to x and reverse the order of differentiation, we obtain

$$\frac{\partial}{\partial x}\left(\frac{\partial F}{\partial t}\right) = \frac{\partial}{\partial t}\underbrace{\left(\frac{\partial F}{\partial x}\right)}_{= f} = \frac{\partial f}{\partial t} = D \frac{\partial^2 f}{\partial x^2} \tag{1.3}$$

Equation (1.3) is the most basic form of the diffusion equation which relates changes of concentration in time and space.

The diffusion equation (1.3) is a partial differential equation in the variables x and t. Clearly, *deriving* such equations from substantive assumptions, such as Fick's, is different from *solving* them. Fortunately, solving partial differential equations is a well-investigated area so that we can often draw on this knowledge to find explicit solutions $f(x, t)$ satisfying a given diffusion equation under the appropriate initial and boundary conditions.

Even so, some qualitative consequences of Eq. (1.3) for simple diffusion processes are immediate. For example, let us assume that at some time t, the concentration f is strictly linear in x in some interval $[a, b]$, that is, $f(x, t) = ux + k$, say. Then the second derivative of f with respect to x will be equal to zero in this interval. According to Eq. (1.3), the density f will then not change with time.

One way to understand that statement is as follows. Fick's assumption (ii) states that the net flow at some inner point x in the interval $[a, b]$ during $[t, t + \Delta t]$ is equal to $-D\frac{\partial f}{\partial x} \Delta t$. Now, if f in $[a, b]$ is linear in x, then $\frac{\partial f}{\partial x} = u$, where u is the (constant) slope of f with respect to x. According to Fick's assumption (ii), this means that the net flow (from left to right) at $x - \Delta x/2$ is $-Du\Delta t$. Similarly, the net flow (from left to right) at $x + \Delta x/2$ is equally $-Du\Delta t$. That is, the inflow at the left border $x - \Delta x/2$ is equal to the outflow at the right border $x + \Delta x/2$, which means that the density f does not change during $[t, t + \Delta t]$. This argument holds for any $[t, t + \Delta t]$; therefore, the concentration f will remain unchanged as long as f is linear in x.

By a similar argument, suppose f is convex in $[a, b]$, so that the first derivative of f with respect to x is increasing in the spatial variable x. Consider again the small interval $[x - \Delta x/2, x + \Delta x/2]$ in $[a, b]$, and suppose that $\frac{\partial f}{\partial x}$ is equal to u at $x - \Delta x/2$. Similarly, $\frac{\partial f}{\partial x}$ will be equal to, say, $u + v$ at $x + \Delta x/2$. If f is convex, then $\frac{\partial f}{\partial x}$ increases, and we must have that $v > 0$, whereas u may be any number. According to Fick's assumption (ii), the difference of inflow at $x - \Delta x/2$ and outflow at $x + \Delta x/2$ will then be $-D[u - (u + v)] \Delta t = Dv\Delta t > 0$. This means that if f is convex, then the local concentration f at x in $[a, b]$ will increase during the short time interval considered. This is exactly what the diffusion Eq. (1.3) expresses because if f is convex, then $\frac{\partial^2 f}{\partial x^2} > 0$. A converse statement holds when f is concave in $[a, b]$, in which case the local concentration f at all x in $[a, b]$ will decrease.

1.3 Exercises

1. Consider the Galton board with four rows shown in Fig. 1.3. What is the probability that two balls end up in the same bin at the bottom? What is the probability that on its way downward a ball is never to the right of its starting point?
2. Suppose you intend to purchase a mechanical Galton board with four rows as shown in Fig. 1.3. To test its construction, you run 1000 balls through the board. How many balls would you expect to end up in the middle bin? What are the upper and lower limits for this number beyond which you would refrain from buying the apparatus?

3. It is sometimes argued that "in the long run chance effects tend to balance out and cancel". Does this mean that in a Galton board with 40 rows the probability for a ball to end in the middle bin right below its starting point is larger than for the board with 4 rows shown in Fig. 1.3?

4. Verify that the normal density with mean zero and variance $\sigma^2 t$

$$f(x, t) = \frac{1}{\sigma\sqrt{2\pi t}} \exp\left(-\frac{x^2}{2\sigma^2 t}\right)$$

is one solution of Eq. (1.3); its diffusion coefficient is $D = \frac{1}{2}\sigma^2$. Investigate the behavior of $f(x, t)$ as $t \to 0$ and also as $t \to \infty$.

5. Give a qualitative argument why for any fixed value of x, the function $f(x, t)$ in Exercise 4 must be first increasing, then reach a maximum, and finally decrease as t increases from $t = 0$ on. Verify this argument formally by investigating $f(x, t)$ for some fixed x as a function of t. Use Eq. (1.3) to explain why the location of the maximum of f w.r.t. t for a given, fixed x also follows from the location of the points of inflection of f w.r.t. x for a given, fixed t.

6. One might be tempted to think that one implication of Eq. (1.3) runs as follows: if for some t the density (concentration) f has a point of inflection at x (so that the second derivative of f w.r.t. x is zero there), then, because $\frac{\partial f}{\partial t} = D \frac{\partial^2 f}{\partial x^2}$, the density at this point will not change any more with t. Explain why this argument is wrong. To this end, consider the solution of Eq. (1.3) in Exercise 4 whose points of inflection are located at $x = \pm\sigma\sqrt{t}$.

7. Verify that for some combinations of α and β, the function

$$f(x, t) = \exp(\alpha x + \beta t)$$

is another solution of Eq. (1.3). Determine its diffusion coefficient D in terms of α and β. Discuss why the function f does not represent an adequate description of the process illustrated in Fig. 1.5. Which conditions on f and which further specifications, in addition to Eq. (1.3), are needed to obtain an adequate solution of the diffusion equation?

Chapter 2
Discrete Random Walks

2.1 The Symmetric Simple Random Walk

The symmetric simple random walk is to diffusion theory what the fruit fly *Drosophila melanogaster* is for genetics: an austere and highly simplified yet non-trivial model case. It is an ideal showpiece that permits us to study several basic conceptual ideas and techniques in their most elementary, purest form to which we can then add more complex generalizations.

Let us consider, then, the movement of a walk that is discrete in both time and space. It starts at position 0 and at any step moves with equal probability (i.e., $p = \frac{1}{2}$) one spatial unit to the left or right; successive steps are independent. Clearly, these assumptions formalize the basic mechanism underlying Galton's board in Fig. 1.3. A typical realization of this process is depicted in Fig. 2.1 which shows the first 100 steps of one realization of a symmetric simple random walk.

The word *simple* in the section title indicates that from any position, the walk can step only to its adjacent positions to the left and right, and the word *symmetric* means that in each step, either of these steps occurs with equal probability. Clearly, both of these aspects are capable of considerable generalizations. For example, in a slightly more general scenario, we might assume that the size of each step equals $\pm\Delta x$ and that the time between any two steps is Δt. We will consider this scenario in Chap. 3 with a view to what happens if both of these quantities tend to zero, in such a way that in the limit a continuous process results. As we will then see, basic results obtained in the present chapter either hold analogously or are modified in rather obvious ways.

© Springer Nature Switzerland AG 2022
W. Schwarz, *Random Walk and Diffusion Models*,
https://doi.org/10.1007/978-3-031-12100-5_2

Fig. 2.1 A typical realization of the first 100 steps of a symmetric simple random walk $\{\mathbf{S}_n, n \geq 1\}$ in which each single step $\mathbf{X}_i$ has size $\Delta x = \pm 1$ and is independent of the past history of the process. The inter-step duration is equal to $\Delta t = 1$. The starting point of the walk is $\mathbf{S}_0 = 0$, and its position after n steps equals $\mathbf{S}_n = \sum_{i=1}^{n} \mathbf{X}_i$. Abscissa, number $n = 1, \ldots$ of step; ordinate, position $\mathbf{S}_n$ after $n \geq 1$ steps

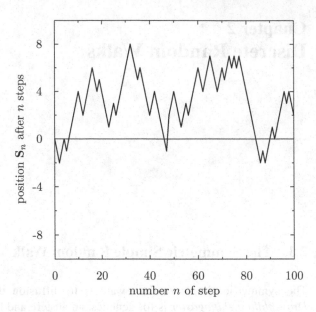

2.1.1   Unrestricted Evolution: Some Basic Properties

The movements of the walk are really the same as that of a ball passing through Galton's board (Sect. 1.2.1). How can we follow and describe the evolution of this simple process? After the first step, the walk will, with equal probability, occupy either position $+1$ or -1. But what about the position after, say, 100 steps? In the extreme, the walk may move to position -100 or $+100$, but just as with Galton's board, there exist many paths leading to middle positions, whereas there is only one path leading to $+100$.

Let the *independent* random variables $\mathbf{X}_i$, $i \geq 1$ denote the size of the i–th step, that is, the displacement of the walk arising with that step. Then $\mathbf{X}_i = \pm 1$ with equal probability. The basic construction is that the position of the walk after n steps is equal to the sum $\mathbf{S}_n = \sum_{i=1}^{n} \mathbf{X}_i$. The entire walk may then be summarized by the successive positions that it had reached after n steps, that is, as $\{\mathbf{S}_n, n \geq 1\}$.

Note that $\mathbf{X}_{n+1}$ is independent of $\mathbf{S}_n$ because the underlying basic random variables $\mathbf{X}_i$ are independent. This means that the next step, $\mathbf{X}_{n+1}$, is independent of the current position, $\mathbf{S}_n$, and also independent of the way in which that position was reached. This property implies that the distribution of $\mathbf{S}_{n+1}$ depends only on $\mathbf{S}_n$ but not on the way in which that position after n steps was reached, the so-called Markovian property. Loosely speaking, according to this property, the future of the process ($\mathbf{S}_{n+1}$) depends only on the present state ($\mathbf{S}_n$) and is independent of the past, that is, of the way in which the present state was reached. In Sect. 2.4, we will consider a modified type of random walk for which these strong assumptions of independence are relaxed. As we will then see, dropping the assumption of independent steps can have quite drastic consequences on the behavior of the associated random walk.

Clearly, in the simple symmetric random walk, we have $E[X_i] = 0$ and so $Var[X_i] = E[X_i^2] = 1$. The implied property that $E[S_n] = 0$ holds even for dependent steps, but when the steps X_i are assumed independently, we also have $Var[S_n] = n$.

As the position after n steps is a sum of independent random variables, by the central limit theorem, we expect it for intermediate and large n to be approximately normal, with mean $\mu = 0$ and variance n. For example, we would expect that if we simulate the first $n = 100$ steps of a great number of simple symmetric random walks, then about 95% of them should have their end positions S_{100} in the interval $[-20, +20]$. These facts will be made more explicit in the slightly more general scenario used in Chap. 3.

2.2 The Simple Random Walk with Drift

2.2.1 Unrestricted Evolution: Some Basic Properties

What changes in the scenario discussed in Sect. 2.1 when $p \neq \frac{1}{2}$? As discussed in Sect. 1.2.1 for the case of Galton's board, the walk will then exhibit a constant tendency—a *drift*—to move upward if $p > \frac{1}{2}$ or downward if $p < \frac{1}{2}$.

To make this notion more precise, the key concept is that each individual step will then with probability p lead to a displacement of $X_i = +1$ and with probability $1 - p$ to a displacement of $X_i = -1$. Thus, the expected displacement in any single step is $(+1) \cdot p + (-1) \cdot (1 - p) = 2p - 1$. Also, the squared displacement always equals $+1$; therefore, the variance of the displacement in any single step is $1 - (2p - 1)^2 = 4p(1 - p)$.

As in the case of $p = \frac{1}{2}$, the position of the walk after n steps is still given by the cumulated successive displacements, that is, by the sum $S_n = \sum_{i=1}^{n} X_i$. In the presence of drift, this implies that

$$E[S_n] = n(2p - 1) \tag{2.1}$$

and from the assumed independence of the steps, we also have

$$Var[S_n] = 4np(1 - p) \tag{2.2}$$

This means that the expected position and the variance of the walk both increase linearly with the number of steps, that is, with time, when the step duration is constant.

To illustrate these results, when $p = 0.501$, then across many independent realizations after $n = 10,000$ steps, the average position of the walk will be 20.

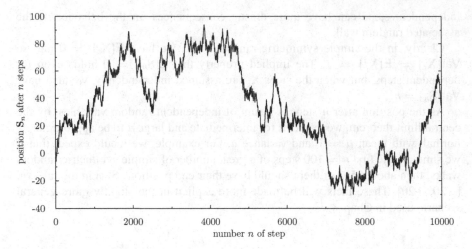

Fig. 2.2 A typical realization of the first 10,000 steps of a simple random walk with a small drift, $p = 0.501$. The maximal height reached is 94, the lowest position is -30; the final level after 10,000 steps is 34. Abscissa, number $n = 1, 2, \ldots$ of step; ordinate, position S_n after $n \geq 1$ steps

Note that this result refers to the walk's average position after a fixed number of exactly 10,000 steps. Even when the expected position increases linearly with the number of steps, this position will in any individual realization of the walk (see Fig. 2.2) typically not be the maximum height that had been reached during these 10,000 steps. Indeed, in Sect. 3.4 and in Exercise 14 of Chap. 4, we will see that on average the maximum height that a walk with $p = 0.501$ reaches within these 10,000 steps is quite a bit higher, about 90. This fits in with the fact that the standard deviation of the walk's position after 10,000 steps is quite large, roughly 100. From the central limit theorem, we expect that after $n = 10,000$ steps, about 95% of all realizations of the walk will be found in the wide interval $20 \pm 2 \cdot 100$, that is, roughly between -180 and 220.

One typical realization of this process is shown in Fig. 2.2; its maximal and minimal height are 94 and -30, respectively, and the final position after 10,000 steps is 34. Note that with the scaling of the axes required by the large number of steps, the process looks much smoother than the one depicted in Fig. 2.1.

2.2.2 The Forward and the Backward Equation

In many contexts, it seems natural to denote the starting point of a random walk as 0, but we will see that a more flexible conceptualization is to view the starting state as another variable, say k, characterizing the process. Starting from an initial state k, a basic quantity of interest for a simple random walk is the probability $p(k, m, n)$ of being—not necessarily for the first time, of course—at state m after exactly n

steps. Similar to the example based on $k = 0$ shown in Fig. 2.1, any individual realization of a random walk can then be thought of as one specific path leading from the starting coordinate $(0|k)$ to the final position $(n|m)$. For fixed values of k and n, we may think of $p(k, m, n)$ as a probability distribution in the variable m— the distribution of states which the walk, starting at k, occupies after n steps. Given that the walk must occupy *some* state after n steps, it must for all n be the case for any fixed k that $p(k, m, n)$ sums to 1 across m.

To derive an equation for $p(k, m, n)$, we partition the set of all paths leading from $(0|k)$ to $(n|m)$ into two mutually exclusive and exhaustive subsets. In fact, we will consider two different such partitions, leading to two separate equations both characterizing the function $p(k, m, n)$.

First, in order to arrive with step n at state m, it is necessarily the case that after $n - 1$ steps, the walk occupies either state $m - 1$ or state $m + 1$. The probability of the first event is by definition $p(k, m - 1, n - 1)$; that of the second is $p(k, m + 1, n - 1)$. As shown in Fig. 2.3, top panel, only from these two states can the final position m be reached with the last, n-th step. That is, any path leading in n steps to the position m must correspond to exactly one of these two scenarios. Furthermore, these scenarios are mutually exclusive so that their probabilities add. Formally, this decomposition conditions on the size of the *final* step, which is either $+1$ (the first scenario) or -1 (the second scenario). Less formally, if the walk is to reach position m after n steps, the final approach to this position is either from below or from above. As successive

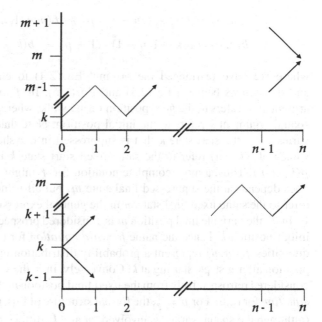

Fig. 2.3 Top panel: Any path from $(0|k)$ to $(n|m)$ must approach the final point either from above or from below; this partition leads to the forward equation (2.3). Bottom panel: The first step of any path from $(0|k)$ to $(n|m)$ must be either upward or downward; this partition leads to the backward equation (2.4). Abscissa, number $n = 0, 1, 2, \ldots$ of step; ordinate, position after $n \geq 0$ steps

steps (specifically, the first $n - 1$ steps and the final, $n-$th step) are independent, we get

$$p(k, m, n) = p(k, m - 1, n - 1) \cdot p + p(k, m + 1, n - 1) \cdot (1 - p) \quad (2.3)$$

An alternative decomposition of $p(k, m, n)$ conditions on the outcome of the *first* step; see Fig. 2.3, bottom panel. Given the size of the first step ($+1$ or -1), there remains the problem to reach, with the $n - 1$ remaining steps, the final position m from the position ($k + 1$ or $k - 1$, respectively) that was reached after the first step. This gives

$$p(k, m, n) = p \cdot p(k + 1, m, n - 1) + (1 - p) \cdot p(k - 1, m, n - 1) \quad (2.4)$$

Both equations have in common that they reduce the $n-$step problem to a problem involving $n - 1$ steps by conditioning on the outcome of one particular step. In Eq. (2.3), this is the final step; in Eq. (2.4), it is the initial step. The equations differ in which of the two spatial variables (the start state k vs. the final state m) remains fixed and which one is varied. In Eq. (2.3), the start state (k) remains the same in all terms on the left-hand and right-hand side, whereas the final state varies (from m to $m \pm 1$). In Eq. (2.4), it is the start state (k) that varies (from k to $k \pm 1$), whereas the final state (m) remains fixed on both sides. If for ease of notation we suppress in each of the two equations the variable that does not change anyway, we get

$$f(m, n) = f(m - 1, n - 1) \cdot p + f(m + 1, n - 1) \cdot (1 - p) \quad (2.5)$$

$$b(k, n) = b(k - 1, n - 1) \cdot (1 - p) + b(k + 1, n - 1) \cdot p \quad (2.6)$$

where we have rearranged the original Eq. (2.4) to emphasize the similarities and differences between Eq. (2.5) and Eq. (2.6). In $f(m, n)$, the variable spatial argument m refers to the *final* position of the walk, whereas in $b(k, n)$, the variable spatial argument k refers to the initial position. Note that f does depend on (i.e., varies with) the start state k that is suppressed in our short notation; however, all values of $f(m, n)$ refer to the same fixed start state k in the general expression $p(k, m, n)$. Thus, a more complete notation for f might be $f_k(m, n)$. Similarly, b does depend on the suppressed final state m, but all values of $b(k, n) = b_m(k, n)$ refer to the same fixed final state m in the general expression $p(k, m, n)$.

In f, the variable final position m is considered prospectively from a given, fixed initial position k, hence the name *forward equation* for (2.5). For any fixed n, the quantities $f_k(m, n)$ represent a probability distribution in the variable m, the final position after n steps, starting at k. Conversely, in b, the variable initial position k is considered retrospectively from the fixed final position m, hence the name backward *equation* for (2.6). For $p = \frac{1}{2}$, the formal structure of Eqs. (2.5) and (2.6) is identical (although the spatial variables involved, m and k, differ), but for $p \neq \frac{1}{2}$, it is not.

Using either equation with the initial (i.e., for $n = 0$) condition $f_k(k, 0) = b_m(m, 0) = 1$, and $f = b = 0$ elsewhere, it is easy to compute recursively any desired probability $p(k, m, n)$. For example, how likely is it that a walk with $p = 0.6$ starting at position $k = 12$ is after $n = 10$ steps at position $m = 16$? Using either Eq. (2.5) or Eq. (2.6), we find that numerically $p(12, 16, 10) = f_{12}(16, 10) = b_{16}(12, 10) = 0.215$.

For the simple random walk, it is not difficult to use a direct combinatorial argument to find the explicit solution for $p(k, m, n)$. Denote as x and y the number of upward and downward steps, respectively, of a path involving n steps. Clearly, then, $x + y = n$. Further, for the walk to move in n steps from k to m, it must also be the case that the net displacement, that is, the difference between the final level and the initial level must be equal to the difference between the number of upward steps and the number of downward steps, which means that $m - k = x - y$. Together, we then get $x = (n + m - k)/2$ and $y = (n - m + k)/2$, the order of the up and down steps being arbitrary. Thus, we must have that

$$p(k, m, n) = \binom{x + y}{x} p^x (1 - p)^y \qquad (2.7)$$

$$\text{where} \quad x = \frac{n + m - k}{2} \quad , \quad y = \frac{n - m + k}{2}$$

and $p(k, m, n) = 0$ if x and y are not nonnegative integers. It is easy to verify that Eq. (2.7) satisfies both the forward Eq. (2.3) and the backward Eq. (2.4). Note that for a given number n of steps $p(k, m, n)$ depends only on the net displacement $m - k = x - y$ of the walk during its n steps, as would be expected from the fact that p is the same at all positions of the walk. For example, the probability to move in 10 steps from 0 to 4 is the same as that of moving in 10 steps from 12 to 16.

In our numerical example, the net displacement from $k = 12$ to $m = 16$ is equal to 4. Thus, of the walk's $n = 10$ steps, $x = 7$ steps must be upward and $y = 3$ downward, in some arbitrary order, giving a net displacement of 4. This means that $p(12, 16, 10)$ is equal to $\binom{10}{7}(0.6)^7(0.4)^3$ or 0.215.

2.3 Discrete Random Walks in the Presence of Barriers

2.3.1 Absorption Probability with a Single Barrier

In some applications, such as Przibram's (1913) classic study described in Sect. 1.1, the main interest centers on the spatio-temporal dynamics of the random walk proper. However, in many contexts, some of which are described in Chap. 7, the underlying random walk as such is *covert*, that is, not directly observable. What in some of these cases is accessible to observation are the event of reaching a critical (e.g., threshold-like) state and the moment when that state is first reached. In this situation, questions of major interest are: how likely is it that a simple random walk will ever reach a given critical state, and if it does, how long will it on average take

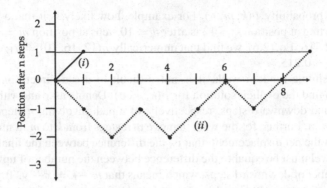

Fig. 2.4 A simple random walk in the presence of an absorbing barrier (horizontal line) at $a = 1$. The first step of the path (full line) labeled (i) is upward so that this path absorbs at $a = 1$ right in the first step. When the first step is downward (dotted line), as in (ii), the path needs to reach, successively, the level 0 and then from there the level $+1$. In the example shown, the path (ii) needs a total of nine steps to reach $a = 1$; after the first downward step, it takes five steps to regain the level 0 and from there another three steps to reach the level 1. Abscissa, number $n = 0, 1, 2, \ldots$ of step; ordinate, position after $n \geq 0$ steps

to reach that level? A related question is: will a simple random walk ultimately reach *any* position, if only it carries on long enough?

To address these questions, let $\lambda(p|a)$ be the probability for a simple random starting at 0 to absorb at—that is, ever reach—the level $a > 0$ when each step is equal to ± 1 with probabilities p and $1 - p$.

For this *one-barrier problem*, we first consider the case of $a = 1$ and seek an equation for $\lambda(p|1)$. As shown in Fig. 2.4, conditioning on the two possible outcomes of the first step, either $a = 1$ is reached directly with that first step (probability p), or else the first step takes the random walk to position -1 (probability $1 - p$). In the latter case, it needs to reach, successively, the level 0 and then from there the level $+1$. These last two passages (getting from -1 to 0 and then from 0 to $+1$) are independent, and from the homogeneity of the simple random walk in time and in its state space, each of them has probability $\lambda(p|1)$. For example, the probability to get back to the level 0 from -1 is $\lambda(p|1)$, the same as reaching the level $+1$ from the start at 0. This gives us the relation

$$\lambda(p|1) = p + (1 - p) \cdot [\lambda(p|1)]^2 \qquad (2.8)$$

which is a quadratic equation in $\lambda(p|1)$ with the two solutions

$$\lambda(p|1) = 1 \qquad \text{and} \qquad \lambda(p|1) = \frac{p}{1 - p} = \varrho$$

where for short we have put ϱ for the odds $\frac{p}{1-p}$ to move upward vs. downward in a single step.

Fig. 2.5 The two solutions of the quadratic equation (2.8). If we require the solution to vary continuously in p and to satisfy the boundary conditions $\lambda(0|1) = 0$ and $\lambda(1|1) = 1$, then we must choose $\lambda(p|1) = \frac{p}{1-p}$ (the increasing curve) in $[0, \frac{1}{2}]$ and $\lambda(p|1) = 1$ (the horizontal curve) in $[\frac{1}{2}, 1]$. For $\frac{1}{2} \leq p \leq 1$, it is certain that the walk will eventually reach the level $a = 1$, whereas for $0 \leq p \leq \frac{1}{2}$, this probability equals $\varrho = \frac{p}{1-p}$

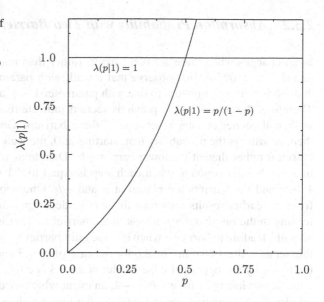

If we require the solution to vary continuously in p and to satisfy the obvious boundary conditions $\lambda(0|1) = 0$ and $\lambda(1|1) = 1$, then Fig. 2.5 shows that the solution is

$$\lambda(p|1) = \begin{cases} \varrho & 0 \leq p \leq \frac{1}{2} \\ 1 & \frac{1}{2} \leq p \leq 1 \end{cases}$$

For example, for $p = \frac{2}{3}$, the probability is 1 that the walk will eventually reach the level $a = 1$, whereas for $p = \frac{1}{3}$, it is only $\frac{1}{2}$.

A barrier at $a > 1$ can only be reached by a successive independent passages from $i - 1$ to i (for $i = 1, \ldots, a$). Reasoning as we did before to derive Eq. (2.8), we get for $a \geq 1$

$$\lambda(p|a) = [\lambda(p|1)]^a = \begin{cases} \varrho^a & 0 \leq p \leq \frac{1}{2} \\ 1 & \frac{1}{2} \leq p \leq 1 \end{cases} \tag{2.9}$$

Thus, for $p \geq \frac{1}{2}$, it is certain that the walk will reach any level $a > 0$ sooner or later, whereas for $p < \frac{1}{2}$, there is a nonzero probability (i.e., $1 - \varrho^a$) that the walk will never reach the level $a > 0$.

2.3.2 Absorption Probability with Two Barriers

What changes when there are two barriers rather than one, say, one at $a > 0$ and one at $-b < 0$? We first observe that a walk with parameter p and barriers at a and $-b$ is mirror-symmetric to one with parameter $1 - p$ and barriers at b and $-a$. Therefore, the results of the previous section indicate that with probability 1, the walk will sooner or later reach one of these barriers. One basic question to ask, then, is: what is the probability that, starting at 0, the walk will absorb at the upper barrier a rather than at the lower barrier $-b$? Denote as $\psi(p|a, b)$ this probability in a *two-barrier problem* when each step is equal to ± 1 with probabilities p and $1 - p$ and the barriers are placed at a and $-b$. One approach to find $\psi(p|a, b)$ from our earlier results rests on a disjunctive decomposition of the set of all paths leading in the *one-barrier problem* to the barrier a. That is, we consider the set of all paths leading to barrier a when a is the only barrier present. We then decompose this set as is illustrated in Fig. 2.6 for the case of $a = 3$ and $b = 4$. As indicated in the figure by the upper path, the barrier at $a = 3$ is either reached directly, that is, without previously visiting $-b = -4$, an event which by definition has probability $\psi(p|a, b)$. Alternatively, as indicated by the lower path in Fig. 2.6, there is at least one visit to $-b$ before reaching a; clearly, this event has probability $1 - \psi(p|a, b)$. In this latter case, upon reaching $-b$, in order to get to the upper barrier a, a remaining distance of $a + b = 7$ needs to be traversed upward; this event has probability $\lambda(p|a + b)$. These two scenarios are mutually exclusive, so that their probabilities

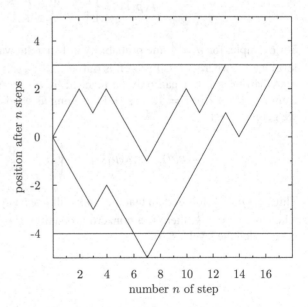

Fig. 2.6 A decomposition to find $\psi(p|a, b)$, for $a = 3$ and $b = 4$. All paths leading to $a = 3$ reach that level either directly (the upper path), that is, without previously visiting $-b = -4$, or else (the lower path) by at least one previous visit to $-b = -4$. In this latter case, a remaining distance of $a + b = 7$ must be traversed upward to reach $a = 3$. Abscissa, number $n = 0, 1, 2, \ldots$ of step; ordinate, position after $n \geq 0$ steps

add, and they are also exhaustive, so that their probabilities sum up to $\lambda(p|a)$. Thus, we must have that

$$\lambda(p|a) = \psi(p|a, b) + [1 - \psi(p|a, b)] \cdot \lambda(p|a + b) \tag{2.10}$$

Formally, the relation Eq. (2.10) is valid for all p, but in view of Eq. (2.9), it is non-trivial only for $0 \leq p < \frac{1}{2}$. Solving Eq. (2.10) for $\psi(p|a, b)$, we get for $0 \leq p < \frac{1}{2}$ the relation

$$\psi(p|a, b) = \frac{\lambda(p|a) - \lambda(p|a + b)}{1 - \lambda(p|a + b)} \tag{2.11}$$

To address the remaining case of $\frac{1}{2} < p \leq 1$, we now use the evident symmetry relation discussed above

$$\psi(p|a, b) = 1 - \psi(1 - p|b, a) \tag{2.12}$$

In both cases, we obtain, on setting $\eta = 1/\varrho = (1 - p)/p$,

$$\psi(p|a, b) = \frac{1 - \eta^b}{1 - \eta^{a+b}} \tag{2.13}$$

The case of $p = \frac{1}{2}$ may now be found from the limit of Eq. (2.13) as $p \rightarrow \frac{1}{2}$:

$$\psi(p|a, b) = \frac{b}{a + b} \quad \text{for} \quad p = \frac{1}{2} \tag{2.14}$$

Another special case results when the barriers are equally distant from the starting point. Inserting $a = b$ into Eq. (2.13), we get the "logistic" probability

$$\psi(p|a, a) = \frac{1}{1 + \eta^a} \tag{2.15}$$

2.3.3   Mean First-Passage Time to a Single Barrier

Next we consider the expected number of steps that a simple random walk needs to reach a for the first time. Across many realizations, this number is clearly a random variable, say $\mathbf{N}$, and is called the first-passage time to the single barrier at $a > 0$. As before, we assume that the walk starts at 0 and that each step is equal to ± 1 with probabilities p and $1 - p$. We will first restrict our analysis to the case $p > \frac{1}{2}$ and denote as $U(a|p) = \mathsf{E}[\mathbf{N}]$ the expected mean first-passage time to the level a.

The expected displacement resulting from any single step equals

$$\mu = \mathsf{E}[\mathbf{X}_i] = (+1) \cdot p + (-1) \cdot (1 - p) = 2p - 1 \qquad (2.16)$$

We know from Eq. (2.9) that for $p > \frac{1}{2}$, it is certain (the probability is 1) that the walk will ultimately reach any level $a \geq 1$. As we reasoned above to obtain Eq. (2.9), the first passage to a consists of the sum of a successive first passages from level $i - 1$ to level i for $i = 1, \ldots, a$, which implies

$$U(a|p) = a \cdot U(1|p) \qquad (2.17)$$

In particular, for $a = 2$, we have

$$U(2|p) = 2 \cdot U(1|p)$$

We next consider the specific case $a = 1$ and again condition on the outcome of the first step; see Fig. 2.4. If the first step $\mathbf{X}_1 = +1$, then evidently $\mathbf{N} = 1$; this event has probability p. With the complementary probability $1 - p$, the first step equals $\mathbf{X}_1 = -1$. In this case, the first passage to $a = 1$ consists of this first step, plus the time needed from level -1 to reach level $+1$, which in view of Eq. (2.17) is in expectation equal to $U(2|p)$. This gives us the relation

$$U(1|p) = p \cdot 1 + (1 - p) \cdot [1 + U(2|p)] = 1 + (1 - p) \cdot U(2|p) \quad , \text{ or}$$

$$U(2|p) = \frac{U(1|p) - 1}{1 - p}$$

On the other hand, we also note from Eq. (2.17) that $U(2|p) = 2 \cdot U(1|p)$, so that

$$U(2|p) = 2 \cdot U(1|p) = \frac{U(1|p) - 1}{1 - p}$$

$$U(1|p) = \frac{1}{2p - 1} = \frac{1}{\mu}$$

and thus for general a and $p > \frac{1}{2}$

$$U(a|p) = a \cdot U(1|p) = \frac{a}{2p - 1} = \frac{a}{\mu} \qquad (2.18)$$

Thus, the mean number of steps needed to reach the level a for the first time is proportional to the distance of that level from the starting point and inversely proportional to the average size of any individual step of the random walk.

What happens to Eq. (2.18) if $p < \frac{1}{2}$ or equivalently if $p > \frac{1}{2}$ but the barrier is *below* the starting point (consider, e.g., a walk with $p = 0.3$ to the level $a = 3$ and one with $p = 0.7$ to the level $b = -3$)? From Eq. (2.9), we know that in this case, the barrier $a > 0$ is reached only with probability $\varrho^a < 1$, whereas with probability

$1 - \varrho^a > 0$, it is never reached at all. This means that for $p < \frac{1}{2}$, the unconditional expectation of **N** is not finite. However, using similar arguments as above, it may be shown (see Exercise 4) that the *conditional* expectation of the number of steps needed to reach a, given that it is ever reached at all, is still given by an expression like Eq. (2.18) but replacing $\mu = 2p - 1$ (which for $p < \frac{1}{2}$ is negative) with $-\mu$, which corresponds to replacing p with $1 - p$.

2.3.4 Mean First-Passage Time with Two Barriers

To extend the result Eq. (2.18), we next consider a random walk starting at 0 between the two barriers a and $-b$ (where $a, b > 0$) and define as $V(a, b|p)$ the expected number of steps needed until the walk reaches either the level a or the level $-b$ for the first time. We will again first restrict our analysis to the case $p > \frac{1}{2}$ and define the two *conditional* expectations $\mathsf{E}_a = \mathsf{E}_a[\mathbf{N}]$ and $\mathsf{E}_{-b} = \mathsf{E}_{-b}[\mathbf{N}]$. For example, E_a is the expected number of steps to the absorption, given that the absorption occurs at a (rather than at $-b$). Correspondingly, E_{-b} is the expected number of steps to the absorption, given that the absorption occurs at $-b$. Weighting each conditional expectation with its own probability as given by Eq. (2.13), we clearly have

$$V(a, b|p) = \mathsf{E}_a \cdot \psi(p|a, b) + \mathsf{E}_{-b} \cdot [1 - \psi(p|a, b)] \qquad (2.19)$$

Reconsidering for a moment the random walk with only a *single* barrier at a, we again use the decomposition argument that was illustrated in Fig. 2.6. That is, all paths ending at a lead either directly—that is, without ever previously visiting $-b$ before—to a or by visiting $-b$ at least once before reaching a.

In the first case, which has probability $\psi(p|a, b)$, the mean duration to reach a is by definition E_a; this case is represented by the left upper limb in Fig. 2.7. In the

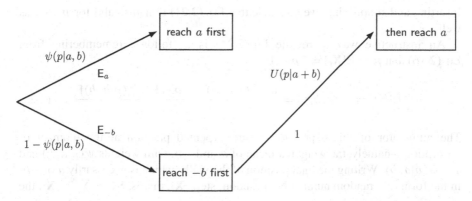

Fig. 2.7 As illustrated in Fig. 2.6, any path starting at 0 first reaches either a (left upper limb) or $-b$ (left lower limb). If $p > \frac{1}{2}$, then with probability 1, paths in the latter class will ultimately reach a from $-b$ (right upward limb); this requires on average $U(a + b|p) = (a + b)/\mu$ additional steps

latter case (probability $1 - \psi(p|a, b)$), after reaching $-b$ which takes on average E_{-b} steps, the walk must then in addition traverse a distance of $a + b$ upward from $-b$ to absorb at a. For $p > \frac{1}{2}$, we know from Eq. (2.9) that this last event (i.e., reaching a from $-b$) has probability 1, and from Eq. (2.18), we know that it takes on average another $U(a + b|p)$ steps. This second scenario is shown in Fig. 2.7 as the left lower plus the right upward limb. Conditioning on these two mutually exclusive and exhaustive cases leading to a, we obtain, using the relation Eq. (2.19), for the mean first-passage time to a single barrier at a

$$U(a|p) = \psi(p|a, b) \cdot E_a + [1 - \psi(p|a, b)] \cdot [E_{-b} + U(a + b|p)]$$

$$= V(a, b|p) + [1 - \psi(p|a, b)] \cdot U(a + b|p) \tag{2.20}$$

We already know the quantities $U(a|p)$, $U(a + b|p)$, and $\psi(p|a, b)$; solving Eq. (2.20) for $V(a, b|p)$ gives

$$\mathbf{E[N]} = V(a, b|p) = U(a|p) - [1 - \psi(p|a, b)] \cdot U(a + b|p)$$

$$= \frac{(a + b) \cdot \psi(p|a, b) - b}{2p - 1}$$

$$= \frac{1}{2p - 1} \cdot \left[(a + b) \cdot \frac{1 - \eta^b}{1 - \eta^{a+b}} - b \right] \tag{2.21}$$

where as before, we have used $\eta = \frac{1-p}{p}$.

We have assumed $p > \frac{1}{2}$ because only then are $U(a|p)$ and $U(a + b|p)$ finite. To get the corresponding results for $p < \frac{1}{2}$ as well, we now employ the evident symmetry relation

$$V(b, a|1 - p) = V(a, b|p)$$

Inserting and simplifying, we conclude that Eq. (2.21) remains valid for $p < \frac{1}{2}$ as well.

An instructive way to rewrite Eq. (2.21) is as follows, remembering from Eq. (2.16) that $\mu = \mathbf{E}[\mathbf{X}_i] = 2p - 1$:

$$\mathbf{E[N]} = V(a, b|p) = \frac{a \cdot \psi(p|a, b) - b \cdot [1 - \psi(p|a, b)]}{\mu} \tag{2.22}$$

The numerator of this expression is the expected position at the moment of absorption—namely, the weighted mean of a and $-b$, with weights $\psi(p|a, b)$ and $1 - \psi(p|a, b)$. Writing the final position of the walk (which is necessarily a or $-b$) in the form of a random number $\mathbf{N}$ of random steps $\mathbf{X}_i$, that is, $\mathbf{S_N} = \sum_{i=1}^{\mathbf{N}} \mathbf{X}_i$, the expected number of steps to absorption is from Eq. (2.22) seen to be

$$E[N] = \frac{E[S_N]}{E[X]} \qquad (2.23)$$

That is, the mean number of steps to absorption is equal to the expected final position, $E[S_N]$, divided by the expected size of a single step, $E[X]$. Or, rearranging Eq. (2.23) into the form of $E[S_N] = E[N] \times E[X]$, we may as well say: the expected final position (which is necessarily the weighted mean of a and $-b$) is equal to the expected number of steps times the mean size of each step.

2.3.5 Conditional Mean First-Passage Time with Two Barriers

The derivations of the previous sections, essentially due to Darling and Siegert (1953), are remarkably effortless and elegant, resting on elementary arguments of representation, path decomposition, and symmetry. A limitation is that they do not immediately produce the separate *conditional* expectations E_a and E_{-b}.

To obtain results for these informative quantities, we need, in addition to Eq. (2.20), a second linearly independent equation involving E_a and E_{-b}, so that we can express the two conditional expectations in terms of known quantities. To this end, Darling and Siegert considered the analogue of Eq. (2.20), again for a *single* barrier, but now for a barrier placed at $-b < 0$ rather than at $a > 0$. Again, we first focus on the case of $p > \frac{1}{2}$.

From symmetry, we know that, for example, for $p = \frac{3}{4}$, the level $-b$ will be reached just as often as the level $+b$ when a single upward step has probability $p' = 1 - p = \frac{1}{4}$. According to Eq. (2.9), for $p > \frac{1}{2}$, the latter probability is equal to

$$\left(\frac{p'}{1-p'}\right)^b = \left(\frac{1-p}{p}\right)^b = \eta^b < 1 \qquad (2.24)$$

That is, when $p > \frac{1}{2}$, only a fraction of η^b of all paths will ever reach the barrier at $-b$ in the one-barrier scenario. However (see Exercise 4), when $p > \frac{1}{2}$, the *conditional* expectation of the number of steps to reach $-b$ for the first time, if it is ever reached at all, is still equal to $U(b|p) = b/\mu$, where as before, the mean step size is $\mu = 2p - 1$.

The basic reasoning to decompose the event of reaching the barrier at $-b$ in the one-barrier scenario is illustrated in Fig. 2.8. One part contributing to the total fraction η^b of all paths ever reaching $-b$ comes from paths which reach $-b$ directly, that is, without ever reaching a before. This component is represented by the left lower limb in Fig. 2.8. This contribution amounts to $1 - \psi(p|a, b)$, and, by definition, the expected number of steps in this case is E_{-b}.

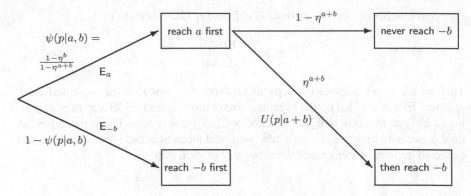

Fig. 2.8 Any path starting at 0 first reaches either a (left upper limb) or $-b$ (left lower limb). With probability η^{a+b} paths in the former class will ultimately reach $-b$ from a (right downward limb); those paths that do reach $-b$ from a will need on average $U(a+b|p) = (a+b)/\mu$ steps. Note that the probability $1 - \eta^b$ of never reaching $-b$ is the product of the conditional probabilities along the two upper limbs, leading up to the event "never reach $-b$"

The second, separate part consists of paths (represented by the left upper limb in Fig. 2.8) which at least once reach a before reaching $-b$ (probability $\psi(p|a, b)$, expected number of steps E_a) and then cross a distance of $a + b$ downward to reach $-b$ from a (the right downward limb in Fig. 2.8). This latter event has probability η^{a+b}, and conditional on ever reaching $-b$ from a the expected number of steps is $U(a + b|p) = (a + b)/\mu$. Taken together, this second part gives a contribution to the overall probability of η^b equal to $\psi(p|a, b) \cdot \eta^{a+b}$, and the expected number of steps in this case is equal to $\mathsf{E}_a + U(a + b|p)$.

Note that the probability weights of $1 - \psi(p|a, b)$ and $\psi(p|a, b) \cdot \eta^{a+b}$ for both scenarios add up to η^b, the total probability of ever reaching the level $-b$. The reason is that the two contributions (the two paths leading to $-b$ in Fig. 2.8) are mutually exclusive and together exhaust the event of ever reaching $-b$ in the one-barrier scenario. Weighting the two means associated with each scenario relative to the overall probability of η^b, this decomposition gives us the relation

$$U(b|p) = \frac{[1 - \psi(p|a, b)] \cdot \mathsf{E}_{-b} + \psi(p|a, b) \cdot \eta^{a+b} \cdot [\mathsf{E}_a + U(a + b|p)]}{\eta^b} \quad (2.25)$$

Together with Eq. (2.20), we have two linearly independent equations for $p > \frac{1}{2}$ which are easily solved for E_a and E_{-b}. The results may be written in the form

$$\mathsf{E}_a[\mathsf{N}] = \frac{1}{\mu} \cdot \left\{ (a + b) \frac{1 + \eta^{a+b}}{1 - \eta^{a+b}} - b \frac{1 + \eta^b}{1 - \eta^b} \right\}$$

$$\mathsf{E}_{-b}[\mathsf{N}] = \frac{1}{\mu} \cdot \left\{ (a + b) \frac{1 + \eta^{a+b}}{1 - \eta^{a+b}} - a \frac{1 + \eta^a}{1 - \eta^a} \right\} \quad (2.26)$$

where as before, $\mu = 2p - 1$ and $\eta = (1 - p)/p$.

By symmetry, a walk with parameters (p, a, b) is the spatial mirror image of a walk characterized by the parameters $(1 - p, b, a)$. Inserting these symmetry relations into Eq. (2.26) shows that the form of E_a and E_{-b} given above remains valid for $p < \frac{1}{2}$ as well.

It is instructive to recover the one-sided mean first-passage times from Eq. (2.26), say, for the case of the upper barrier at a. When $p > \frac{1}{2}$, we have $\eta < 1$ and $\mu > 0$. In this case, E_a in Eq. (2.26) tends to a/μ as $b \to \infty$, in line with our previous result Eq. (2.21). On the other hand, when $p < \frac{1}{2}$, we have $\eta > 1$ and $\mu < 0$. In this case, E_a in Eq. (2.26) tends to $-a/\mu$ as $b \to \infty$. As discussed at the end of Sect. 2.3.3 and in Exercise 4, when $p < \frac{1}{2}$ and there is only a single barrier at $a > 0$, the unconditional mean-first passage time to this barrier is infinite, as the random walk will with probability $1 - \varrho^a$ never reach the barrier at a. However, the conditional mean first-passage time, given the walk does ultimately reach a, is still given by $a/|\mu|$, in analogy to Eq. (2.21).

An instructive way to rewrite the unwieldy Eq. (2.26) more compactly is to define the function $h(t) = (t/\mu) \cdot \coth(kt)$ where coth is the hyperbolic cotangent, $\mu = 2p - 1$, and $k = \frac{1}{2} \ln[p/(1 - p)]$. Then

$$E_a[\mathbf{N}] = h(a + b) - h(b)$$

$$E_{-b}[\mathbf{N}] = h(a + b) - h(a) \tag{2.27}$$

As shown in Fig. 2.9, the function h is increasing ($h' > 0$) and convex ($h'' > 0$). The first property implies that $h(a + b) - h(b)$ increases in a, and the second property implies that it increases in b. Corresponding observations with interchanged roles of a and b can be made for $h(a + b) - h(a)$. Together, they imply that both E_a and E_{-b} increase in a and in b: increasing the distance of either barrier will always lead to increases of both conditional mean first-passage times.

Furthermore, from Eq. (2.27), the difference of the conditional mean first-passage times is clearly

$$E_a[\mathbf{N}] - E_{-b}[\mathbf{N}] = h(a) - h(b) \tag{2.28}$$

As h is increasing, Eq. (2.28) implies that for all values of p, the barrier that is closer to the origin is always associated with the shorter conditional mean first-passage time. In particular, when the barriers are equally distant from the start point, $a = b$, then the conditional mean first-passage times to both barriers are for all values of p identical. For example, for $p = 0.9$ and $a = b$, the walk absorbs much more often at the upper barrier a than at the lower barrier $-a$; however, absorptions at a and at $-a$ take on average the same number of steps. The property is relevant, for example, to the work of Gold and Shadlen (2001), Gold and Shadlen (2007) on models of neuronal activity in perceptual decision-making, presented in Sect. 7.6.1.

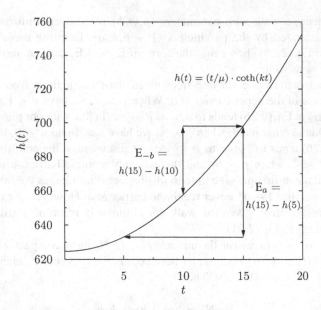

Fig. 2.9 The function $h(t) = (t/\mu) \cdot \coth(kt)$ for $p = 0.52$ so that $\mu = 2p - 1 = 0.040$ and $k = \frac{1}{2}\ln[p/(1 - p)] = 0.040$. For barriers placed at $a = 10$ and $-b = -5$, the conditional mean first-passage times are $E_a = 65.0$ and $E_{-b} = 40.3$. According to Eq. (2.27), these values result as $h(15) - h(5)$ and $h(15) - h(10)$, respectively. As h is increasing and convex, $E_a = h(a+b) - h(b)$ and $E_{-b} = h(a + b) - h(a)$ increase in a and in b. Also, the barrier that is closer to the origin is for all values of p associated with the shorter conditional mean first-passage time

2.3.6 Generating Functions for First-Passage Problems

The arguments illustrated in Fig. 2.4 and leading to Eq. (2.8) can be generalized at little cost but considerable benefit by the use of probability generating functions (pgfs). The pgf of a positive discrete random variable N is defined as

$$g(z) = E[z^N] = \sum_{n=1}^{\infty} z^n \cdot P(N = n) \qquad (2.29)$$

Some properties of g immediately follow from this definition. For example, for any regular (non-defective) distribution, it must be the case that $g(1) = 1$. Furthermore, evaluated at $z = 1$, the derivative $g'(z) = E[Nz^{N-1}]$ of g clearly reduces to the expectation $E[N]$; higher moments are obtained from the higher-order derivatives. Similarly, $g'(z = 0)$ gives $P(N = 1)$, and in principle, the entire probability distribution of N can be recovered from g by evaluating its derivatives at $z = 0$.

A key feature of pgfs that is central for discrete random walks is the convolution property: if N and M are independent discrete random variables, then the pgf of their sum $N + M$ is $E[z^{N+M}] = E[z^N] \cdot E[z^M]$, that is, the product of their individual pgfs.

In particular, if $\mathbf{N}$ and $\mathbf{M}$ are identically distributed, both having pgf g, then the pgf of their sum is equal to g^2. An excellent treatment of pgfs is given by Feller (1968, ch. XI).

We consider a simple discrete random walk with step probability $p > \frac{1}{2}$ starting at 0 and ask for the generating function $g(z)$ of the first-passage time $\mathbf{N}_1$ to the level $a = +1$. As explained in Sect. 2.3.1 and Fig. 2.4, the basic decomposition is to condition on the outcome ($+1$ or -1) of the first step.

Thus, with probability p, the first step leads right to $a = 1$, and then the first-passage time $\mathbf{N}_1$ is simply equal to 1. With probability $1 - p$, the first step leads to the level -1; in this case, the walk has consumed one step and must first reach from -1 the level 0 and then from 0 the level $+1$. This means that with probability $1 - p$, the number of steps to reach the level $a = 1$ is distributed as $1 + \mathbf{N}_1' + \mathbf{N}_1''$ where $\mathbf{N}_1'$ and $\mathbf{N}_1''$ are two independent first-passage times, both distributed as is $\mathbf{N}_1$. Taken together, this decomposition implies that the pgf $g(z)$ of $\mathbf{N}_1$ satisfies

$$\mathsf{E}[z^{\mathbf{N}_1}] = p\,\mathsf{E}[z^1] + (1 - p)\,\mathsf{E}[z^{1+\mathbf{N}_1'+\mathbf{N}_1''}]$$

$$g(z) = pz + (1 - p)\,z\,g(z)\,g(z) \qquad (2.30)$$

Dividing through by $(1 - p)\,z$ and rearranging gives

$$g^2(z) - \frac{1}{(1 - p)z}\,g(z) + \frac{p}{1 - p} = 0$$

This is a quadratic equation in g, and from Eq. (2.9), we know that for $p > \frac{1}{2}$, we must have that $g(1) = 1$. The relevant solution satisfying this condition is

$$g(z) = \frac{1 - \sqrt{1 - 4p(1 - p)z^2}}{2(1 - p)z} \qquad (2.31)$$

We noted above that the first-passage time to a level $a > 0$ is the sum of the successive first passages from level $i - 1$ to level i for $i = 1, \ldots, a$. These a successive first passages are independent and are all distributed as is $\mathbf{N}_1$. Therefore, using the convolution property of the pgf referred to above, the pgf of the first-passage time $\mathbf{N}_a$ through the level a is $[g(z)]^a$, with g given in Eq. (2.31).

Clearly, in contrast to results about probabilities and means, the pgf of $\mathbf{N}_a$ is not a directly relevant quantity in itself. Why, then, should we be interested in this pgf at all? First, we can extract in a standard manner from the pgf directly relevant information about the distribution, the mean, and the variance of $\mathbf{N}_a$; see Exercise 4. Second, using decomposition arguments analogous to those used in Sects. 2.3.2 and 2.3.4, we could derive, for example, the pgf of the first-passage time in the two-barrier scenario from that in the one-barrier scenario. Finally, and perhaps most relevant, we can use the pgf of $\mathbf{N}_a$ in the discrete case to arrive at corresponding results for random walks in which many small steps of short duration tend in the limit to a continuous diffusion process. This latter use of the pgf of N_a will be explained in detail in Sects. 3.3 and 4.2.3.

2.4   The Correlated Random Walk

All considerations in this chapter so far relied on the central assumption that the successive steps of the random walk are independent of each other: the value of step X_i does not influence what the value of step X_{i+1} will be. It is easy to imagine real-world processes in which successive steps will be dependent, as, for example, with the successive steps made by an animal exploring an environment (Fig. 1.1). What changes if this central assumption of independence is incorrect?

In this section, we address this question using what is perhaps the simplest non-trivial version of random walks with dependent steps. The so-called correlated, or persistent, random walk models the kind of systematic persistence that one often sees in processes such as the movement of animals or in the choice behavior of humans. As in the simple random walk, we assume that the individual steps are either $+1$ (upward) or -1 (downward) and that each step takes one time unit. We will see in later chapters that we may relax these assumptions and use steps of size Δx and duration Δt, but to focus on the critical aspect of dependency (or persistence), we will for now use the simpler formulation.

2.4.1   Unrestricted Evolution: The Basic Transition Matrix

The basic assumption of correlated random walks is that the probability of an upward (positive) movement in step number $n + 1$ depends on whether the previous step number n had also been upward or not. More specifically, consider the following matrix of transition probabilities for the individual step sizes:

$$
\mathbf{X}_n \quad
\begin{array}{c}
 \\
- \\
+
\end{array}
\begin{array}{cc}
\quad\;\; - & \quad\;\; + \\
\begin{bmatrix} p & 1-p \\ 1-p & p \end{bmatrix}
\end{array}
\tag{2.32}
$$

$\mathbf{X}_{n+1}$

According to matrix (2.32), the random walk will continue in its direction (persist) with probability p and change directions with probability $1 - p$. Thus, the parameter p models the *persistence* of the walk. It is crucial to realize that its conceptual meaning is quite different from that of p in the simple random walk with independent steps. This is perhaps best seen by considering extreme boundary cases. If $p \to 1$, then the walk converges to pure persistence, and its path forms a deterministic straight line. If $p \to 0$, then it tends to change its direction with every new step, and its path forms a zigzag line in which ups and downs alternate regularly. For $p = 0.5$, we clearly have a symmetric simple random walk with independent steps. As suggested by the symmetry of the transition matrix (2.32), we know from general Markov chain theory (see Ross 2019, ch. 4) that as $n \to \infty$ up and down steps are equally likely and that the long-run proportion of up and down steps tends to $\frac{1}{2}$. In a more general formulation than Eq. (2.32), the probability p of persistence could depend on the value of the previous step (see Sect. 7.4), but for now, we will focus on the simpler symmetric variant.

Our considerations of the limiting case $p \to 1$ emphasize another point that is crucial for correlated random walks, but is absent for simple random walks. Precisely because successive steps are independent in simple random walks, we did not need to consider the *directional state* (i.e., the value of the preceding step) the process is in when it starts. In contrast, to analyze correlated random walks, it is necessary to know if the process is in an upward or downward directional state before the first step is executed.

As indicated at the left vertical axis in Fig. 2.10, we can imagine a hypothetical zero-th step that was upward or downward and then use the transition matrix (2.32) to generate step number 1 and all steps following it. For example, if the zero-th step was upward (the full line in Fig. 2.10), then the first step will be upward with probability p and downward with $1 - p$. Similarly, for $p \to 1$, the walk will tend

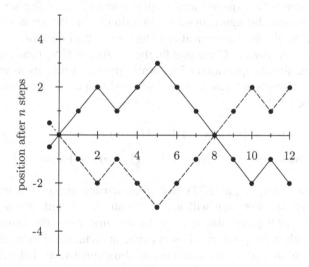

Fig. 2.10 The basic symmetry relation for correlated random walks starting at $x_0 = 0$. Abscissa, number n of steps; ordinate, position of the walk after n steps. As indicated to the left of the vertical axis, the walk shown as a full line starts in the upward directional state; according to matrix (2.32), its successive steps have probabilities $p \cdot p \cdot (1-p) \cdot (1-p) \cdot p \cdot (1-p) \cdot p \cdot p \cdot p \cdot p \cdot (1-p) \cdot (1-p)$. The walk shown as a broken line starts in the downward state and is the mirror image of the full-line walk; its successive step probabilities are identical to that of the walk in full line

to a linear upward movement if it starts in the upward directional state but will tend
to a linear downward movement otherwise. The crucial point here is that without
information about the initial directional state, the transition probabilities for the first
step remain undefined.

Also indicated by the two paths in Fig. 2.10 is a fundamental symmetry property
of correlated random walks. This property follows directly from the transition
matrix (2.32), and we will repeatedly exploit it in the sequel. According to this
property, the mirror image of any given path of a correlated random walk has the
same probability as the original path if its initial directional state is opposite to that
of the original path. For a fixed p, consider the class of all paths starting at $x_0 = 0$
with initial upward directional state and that of all paths starting at $x_0 = 0$ with
initial downward directional state. Because the symmetry property holds for any
path in the (say) first class, the expected position after n steps of walks starting in
the upward directional state must be minus the corresponding expectation for walks
(with the same p) with initial downward directional state; see Fig. 2.10. Similarly,
the expected square of the position of walks in both classes must be the same, and
because the expected positions differ only in sign, the same is true of their variance.

2.4.2 The Mean and Variance of Correlated Random Walks

If $\{\mathbf{X}_i, i \geq 1\}$ are the individual steps of a correlated random walk starting at position
$x_0 = 0$, then what is the expected total displacement of the walk after n steps? As
explained, we need to distinguish in which directional state the process is starting, so
let us denote as $\mathbf{S}_n^+$ the displacement after n steps when the initial direction is upward
and as $\mathbf{S}_n^-$ if it is downward. Correspondingly, let $a(n) = \mathsf{E}[\mathbf{S}_n^+]$ and $b(n) = \mathsf{E}[\mathbf{S}_n^-]$
denote the conditional expectation of the walk given that it starts in an upward or
downward directional state, respectively. We condition on the outcome of the first
step and get the relations

$$a(n) = p \cdot [1 + a(n - 1)] + (1 - p) \cdot [-1 + b(n - 1)] \qquad (2.33)$$

$$b(n) = p \cdot [-1 + b(n - 1)] + (1 - p) \cdot [1 + a(n - 1)] \qquad (2.34)$$

To explain, for example, Eq. (2.33), note that starting at $x_0 = 0$ in an upward
directional state, the first step will lead to position $+1$ with probability p and
to position -1 with probability $1 - p$. In the first case, the expected further
displacement, relative to position $+1$, is in expectation identical to the displacement
in $n - 1$ steps, starting at $x_0 = 0$ in an upward directional state, that is, to $a(n - 1)$.
In the second case, the expected further displacement, relative to position -1, is
in expectation identical to the displacement in $n - 1$ steps, starting at $x_0 = 0$ in a
downward directional state, that is, to $b(n - 1)$.

One way to solve Eqs. 2.33 and 2.34 is to express, say, $b(n)$ in terms of $a(n)$
using Eq. (2.33) and then to insert for $b(n)$ into Eq. (2.34). This approach gives the

second-order equation

$$a(n) - 2p \cdot a(n-1) + (2p-1) \cdot a(n-2) = 0 \tag{2.35}$$

If we put $d(n) = a(n) - a(n-1)$, this equation may be rewritten in terms of $d(n)$ in the more obvious form as

$$d(n) = (2p-1) \cdot d(n-1) \tag{2.36}$$

A somewhat simpler approach is to note the symmetry explained in Fig. 2.10 which means that for every possible full-line path (starting in the upward direction), there is an equally likely broken-line mirror path (starting in the downward direction) whose positions (when the start is at $x_0 = 0$) differ only in their sign. This symmetry implies that $b(n) = -a(n)$, and on inserting into Eq. (2.33), it leads to the simpler first-order equation

$$a(n) = (2p-1) \cdot [1 + a(n-1)] \tag{2.37}$$

The initial conditions are clearly $a(0) = 0$ and $a(1) = 2p - 1$, and the solution satisfying these conditions is

$$a(n) = -b(n) = \frac{2p-1}{2(1-p)} \left[1 - (2p-1)^n \right] \tag{2.38}$$

Figure 2.11 illustrates the typical behavior of $a(n)$ for $n = 6$ steps as a function of the persistence parameter p.

Only for the exceptional cases $p = 0$ (and n even) and $p = 0.5$ (the symmetric simple random walk with independent steps) is $E[S_n^+] = 0$. As observed above, if $p \to 1$, then the walk will simply continue linearly in its initial direction, and then $E[S_n^+] = +n$ and $E[S_n^-] = -n$, depending on the initial directional state. In all intermediate cases, the expected displacement remains bounded and reflects the bias resulting from the initial directional state. Formally, for $0 < p < 1$, the term $(2p-1)^n$ in Eq. (2.38) vanishes for large n, and then the expected displacement of the walk tends to $\pm \frac{2p-1}{2(1-p)}$, the sign depending on the initial directional state. For example, even in a case of very marked persistence as strong as $p = 0.9$, the asymptotic expected displacement as $n \to \infty$ is only ± 4.

As Fig. 2.10 suggests, these results reflect that there is an inherent up-down symmetry in this simplest form of a correlated random walk, persistent movements being equally likely in both directions. The only source of systematically biased displacements is the initial directional state in which the process starts, and this bias converges soon, typically to small values, for any fixed $0 < p < 1$.

Of course, individual realizations of a correlated random walk will fluctuate around the expected value given by Eq. (2.38); to capture this aspect, we next look at the variance of the walk's displacement after n steps. Before doing any actual computations, the variance of S_n may be seen to be independent of the initial

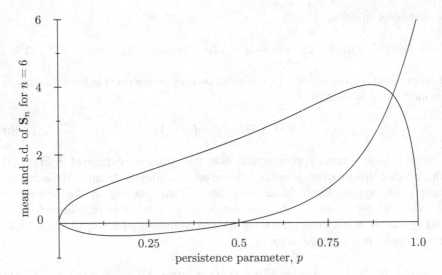

Fig. 2.11 The ordinate shows the mean (the initially decreasing line; $a(n)$ in Eq. (2.38)) and standard deviation (computed from Eq. (2.41)) of the position $\mathbf{S}_n^+$ of a correlated random walk after $n = 6$ steps, as a function of the persistence parameter p (abscissa). The walk starts at position $x_0 = 0$ in an upward directional state. For $p = 0$, the walk always (variance $= 0$) executes six alternating up-and-down steps, returning it to its start position 0. For $p = 1$, the walk always (variance $= 0$) executes six upward steps in sequence, carrying it to position 6. The expected position first decreases in p to a shallow minimum at $p = 0.165$ and then increases. The standard deviation increases to a maximum at $p = 0.871$. At this value, the walk typically persists in its direction, often showing no or only one change of direction during its six steps; this behavior maximizes the standard deviation of the final position $\mathbf{S}_n^+$

directional state, as follows. We first note that $\mathrm{Var}[\mathbf{S}_n] = \mathsf{E}[\mathbf{S}_n^2] - \mathsf{E}^2[\mathbf{S}_n]$, and we already know that $\mathsf{E}[\mathbf{S}_n]$ differs only in sign when starting with different initial directional states, that is, $\mathsf{E}[\mathbf{S}_n^-] = -\mathsf{E}[\mathbf{S}_n^+]$. Therefore, the squared expectation $\mathsf{E}^2[\mathbf{S}_n]$ in the variance expression is independent of the initial directional state. Also, by the symmetry argument illustrated in Fig. 2.10, for any full-line path (i.e., one starting in upward initial direction), there exists a broken-line mirror path (starting in downward initial direction) that has equal probability and whose end position differs only in sign. This implies that the expected square $\mathsf{E}[\mathbf{S}_n^2]$ is the same when starting with initial upward or downward direction, and we denote this common expected square as $c(n)$.

To determine $c(n)$, let us assume that the initial direction is upward; a completely analogous argument holds if it is downward. We again condition on the outcome of the first step. If it is $+1$, which has probability p, then we effectively look for the expectation of $(1 + \mathbf{S}_{n-1}^+)^2$, where as before, $\mathbf{S}_{n-1}^+$ is the displacement after $n-1$ steps when the initial direction is upward; for example, $\mathbf{S}_{n-1}^+$ has expectation $a(n-1)$. Similarly, if the first step is -1, which has probability $1 - p$, then we look for the expectation of $(-1 + \mathbf{S}_{n-1}^-)^2$, where as before, $\mathbf{S}_{n-1}^-$ is the displacement after $n-1$

steps when the initial direction is downward. This approach gives

$$c(n) = \mathsf{E}[S_n^2] = p \cdot \mathsf{E}[(1 + S_{n-1}^+)^2] + (1-p) \cdot \mathsf{E}[(-1 + S_{n-1}^-)^2] \qquad (2.39)$$

Carrying out the squares, noting that $\mathsf{E}[(S_{n-1}^+)^2] = \mathsf{E}[(S_{n-1}^-)^2] = c(n-1)$, and simplifying, we get the recursion

$$c(n) = c(n-1) + 2a(n-1) + 1 \qquad (2.40)$$

where $a(n) = \mathsf{E}[S_n^+]$ is as given by Eq. (2.38). The solution satisfying the initial condition $c(0) = 0$ is

$$\mathsf{E}[S_n^2] = c(n) = \frac{np}{1-p} - \frac{2p-1}{2(1-p)^2}\left[1 - (2p-1)^n\right] \qquad (2.41)$$

The variance of S_n is found as $\mathsf{Var}[S_n] = c(n) - a^2(n)$.

In marked contrast to the means of S_n^+ and S_n^-, their common variance increases with n, in an essentially linear fashion when n is large and $0 < p < 1$. For $p = 0.5$ (the symmetric simple random walk), the variance is equal to n; for $p \to 0$ and $p \to 1$, it necessarily tends to zero. When $n > 1$, the variance is smaller than n for $p < 0.5$ and increases to a maximum in p that is located closer to 1 as n increases. Figure 2.11 illustrates and explains the typical behavior for $n = 6$ steps.

2.4.3 Correlated Random Walks Between Absorbing Barriers

Just as we did for a simple random walk, we may consider correlated random walks between two absorbing barriers. As before, we may then ask how likely it is to absorb at the one or other barrier and how much time it takes on average to reach one of them. To answer these questions, the notation gets slightly more convenient when we assume that the absorbing barriers are placed at $x = 0$ and $x = a$ and that the correlated random walk starts at an intermediate position $0 < r < a$. Of course, the results are then easy to translate into a scenario with barriers at a and $-b$ and a start at 0.

As explained in the previous section, for correlated random walks, we have to take into account the initial directional state in which the process starts. Denote as $u(r)$ the probability to absorb at the upper barrier a when starting at position r if the initial directional state is upward, as illustrated by the full-line path in Fig. 2.12. Similarly, let $v(r)$ denote the probability to absorb at the upper barrier a if the start is at r and the initial directional state is downward; see the broken-line path in

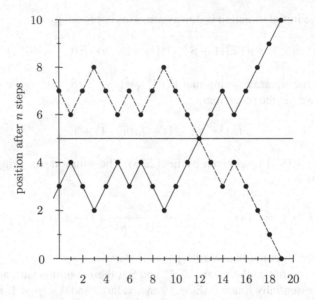

Fig. 2.12 Abscissa, number of step; ordinate, position of the walks after n steps. The full-line path shows a correlated random walk between two absorbing barriers at 0 and $a = 10$; it starts at $r = 3$ in an upward directional state and absorbs after 19 steps at the upper barrier. The broken-line path shows the mirror image of this path, reflected at the black line $y = a/2$; it thus starts at $r = 7$ in a downward directional state. At the moment when the full-line path reaches one of the barriers (here: the upper barrier) for the first time, the broken-line path necessarily reaches the other barrier for the first time. Crucially, both paths have identical probabilities. To any full-line path (starting at $r = 3$ in an upward directional state), there corresponds exactly one broken-line path (starting at $r = 7$ in a downward directional state); their probabilities to absorb at the (say) upper barrier are complementary (they add to 1), and the mean first-passage time to absorption at either barrier is the same

Fig. 2.12. Conditioning on the outcome of the first step, we obtain the equations

$$u(r) = p \cdot u(r+1) + (1-p) \cdot v(r-1) \tag{2.42}$$

$$v(r) = p \cdot v(r-1) + (1-p) \cdot u(r+1) \tag{2.43}$$

Much as with Eqs. (2.33) and (2.34), we may express v in terms of u using Eq. (2.42) and then insert for v into Eq. (2.43). On simplifying, this approach produces the second-order equation

$$u(r) - 2 \cdot u(r-1) + u(r-2) = 0 \tag{2.44}$$

Rewriting Eq. (2.44) in the simpler form of

$$u(r) - u(r-1) = u(r-1) - u(r-2)$$

we see that u increases by the same amount each time its argument increases by one unit. Thus, the general solution for u is a linear function in r, whose intercept and slope depend on p and a. Clearly, $u(a) = 1$, and for $p = 0.5$, we must have that $u(r) = r/a$, the known result Eq. (2.14) for the simple symmetric random walk. The specific solution satisfying these boundary conditions is

$$u(r) = \frac{r + \frac{2p-1}{1-p}}{a + \frac{2p-1}{1-p}} \qquad (2.45)$$

From the relation between $u(r)$ and $v(r)$ expressed in Eq. (2.42), we then get

$$v(r) = \frac{r}{a + \frac{2p-1}{1-p}} \qquad (2.46)$$

Appealing to the symmetry property illustrated in Fig. 2.12, a correlated random walk with initial upward direction starting at r is as likely to absorb at the upper barrier a as is a random walk with initial downward direction starting at $a - r$ is to absorb at the lower barrier 0. This means that $1 - v(a - r) = u(r)$, as is easy to verify from the solutions given. Note that we cannot insert into Eq. (2.45) for $u(r)$ with $r = 0$ as it is impossible to start at the absorbing barrier 0 from an initial upward direction; in contrast, for $r = a$, Eq. (2.45) correctly yields $u(a) = 1$. Similarly, we cannot insert into Eq. (2.46) for $v(r)$ with $r = a$ as it is impossible to start at the absorbing barrier a from an initial downward direction. On forming $u(r) - v(r)$, we can see that the difference resulting from starting at r with upward vs. downward initial direction is independent of r and typically quite small when a is not very small and p not very close to 0 or 1.

How long does it take in expectation until a correlated random walk starting at $0 < r < a$ reaches one of the absorbing barriers? Denote this expectation as $w(r)$ if the walk starts in an upward directional state and as $z(r)$ if it starts in a downward directional state. As indicated in Fig. 2.12, it must then be the case that $z(a - r) = w(r)$.

As before, we condition on the outcome of the first step and obtain

$$w(r) = p \cdot [1 + w(r + 1)] + (1 - p) \cdot [1 + z(r - 1)] \qquad (2.47)$$

$$z(r) = p \cdot [1 + z(r - 1)] + (1 - p) \cdot [1 + w(r + 1)] \qquad (2.48)$$

For example, starting in the upward directional state, with probability p, the first step leads to position $r + 1$, the walk is still in the upward directional state, and one step has been consumed. Similarly, with probability $1 - p$, the first step leads to position $r - 1$, the walk is now in the downward directional state, and one step has been consumed. This explains Eq. (2.47), and Eq. (2.48) is derived analogously. By the same technique used before, we reduce the pair of equations to a single second-order equation. On simplifying, this approach produces

$$w(r) - 2 \cdot w(r-1) + w(r-2) + 2\frac{1-p}{p} = 0 \qquad (2.49)$$

Equation (2.49) implies that the second-order differences in w are constant, which means that w is a quadratic function in r. The solutions satisfying the boundary conditions $w(a) = z(0) = 0$ are

$$w(r) = (a-r) \cdot \left[1 + (r-1) \cdot \left(\frac{1-p}{p} \right) \right] \qquad (2.50)$$

$$z(r) = r \cdot \left[1 + (a-r-1) \cdot \left(\frac{1-p}{p} \right) \right] \qquad (2.51)$$

Figure 2.13 illustrates these results. Note that clearly $w(r) = z(a-r)$, as we would expect from the symmetry property shown in Fig. 2.12. This property implies that,

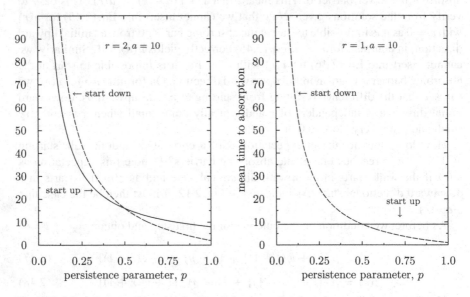

Fig. 2.13 Mean time to absorption (ordinate) for a correlated random walk between absorbing barriers at 0 and $a = 10$ as a function of the persistence parameter, p (abscissa). The walk starts at $r = 2$ (left panel) or at $r = 1$ (right panel), in an upward (full line) or downward (broken line) directional state; see Eqs. (2.50) and (2.51). Both graphs illustrate the case that the start is closer to the lower barrier (i.e., $r < a/2$). For start positions $r > 1$ (left panel), mean time to absorption generally decreases as the walk's persistence increases. For $p > 0.5$, the mean first-passage time is shorter when starting in the downward directional state; as $p \to 1$, the full line necessarily tends to $a - r$ and the broken line to r. For $p < 0.5$, the mean first-passage time is shorter when starting in the upward directional state. When starting in an initial upward directional state at $r = 1$, the mean first-passage time is $a - 1$, independent of p (right panel, full line)

for even a, correlated walks starting at $r = a/2$ will have a mean first-passage time that is independent of the initial directional state, $w(a/2) = z(a/2)$.

For $p = 0.5$, Eqs. (2.50) and (2.51) simplify to $w(r) = z(r) = r \cdot (a - r)$, the known result for simple symmetric random walks (cf., Exercise 1). For $p = 1$, the walk simply continues in its initial direction, giving $w(r) = a - r$ and $z(r) = r$. As $p \rightarrow 0$, the walk tends to alternating up and down steps. Thus, if starting more than one step away from the barriers, the probability tends to 0 that the walk will ever be absorbed, and the expected time to reach one of the boundaries increases beyond any finite limit.

As we would expect, for nearly all starting points r, the mean first-passage time decreases as the persistence parameter p increases: the walk will then approach and reach one of the barriers sooner, without too many time-consuming turns. The cases involving the starting positions $r = 1$ and $r = a - 1$ are special and require some comment, as Eqs. (2.50) and (2.51) simplify to $w(1) = z(a-1) = a-1$ for all values of $0 < p \leq 1$. That is, for these cases, the expected number of steps to absorption is independent of the persistence probability, p.

Consider, for example, a correlated walk that starts in the initial upward directional state at $r = 1$ (the full line in the right panel of Fig. 2.13). Clearly, as $p \rightarrow 1$, it will then take $a - 1$ steps to reach the upper barrier a. In contrast, for, say, $p = 0.01$, the walk will absorb at the lower barrier 0 with probability 0.99 right in the first step. However, in those rare cases when it moves further upward in the first step (i.e., to position 2), it will take a very long time to reach any barrier because the walk will change directions with nearly each step. The result $w(1) = a - 1$ shows that for $r = 1$, probabilities and expected durations balance in a way so that effectively the influence of p cancels.

2.4.4 Correlated Random Walks with Randomized Initial Directional State

In the preceding sections, we have seen that to analyze correlated (persistent) random walks, we need to specify not only the start position of the walk but also the initial directional state (upward or downward). In fact, with the simple model of persistence characterized by Eq. (2.32), this initial directional state is the only source of asymmetric drift-like effects.

A relatively mild generalization of the simplest form of correlated random walks described in Sect. 2.4.1 is to randomize across the initial directional states in which the process starts. To this end, let us indicate the initial directional state by the binary random variable $\mathbf{D}$. Specifically, we let $\mathbf{D} = +1$ if the process starts in the upward directional state and $\mathbf{D} = -1$ if it starts in the downward directional state. We assume that the walk starts with probability $g = P(\mathbf{D} = +1)$ in the upward state and with probability $1 - g$ in the downward state. The expected value of $\mathbf{D}$ is then $2g - 1$, its variance is $4g(1 - g)$, and the two special cases $g = 0$ and $g = 1$ correspond to the fixed initial directional states considered in our analyses so far.

As for the expected displacement after n steps, we must then have that

$$E[S_n] = E[E[S_n|D]] \tag{2.52}$$

where the outer expectation refers to the random variable D and the inner conditional expectation to the random variable S_n, given the initial directional state, that is, given the variable D. As we have seen (cf., Eq. (2.38)), the initial directional state only changes the sign of the expected position, which means that we may write

$$E[S_n|D] = D \cdot a(n)$$

where $a(n)$ is given by Eq. (2.38). Therefore, we also have

$$E[S_n] = E[D \cdot a(n)] = (2g - 1) \cdot a(n) \tag{2.53}$$

In particular, if the process starts with equal probability (i.e., $g = \frac{1}{2}$) in an upward or downward directional state, then the expectation of S_n will be zero for all p and all n. This is a direct consequence of the symmetry property explained in Fig. 2.10. Our previous results Eq. (2.38) for $a(n)$ and $b(n) = -a(n)$ appear as the special cases of Eq. (2.53) when $g = 1$ and $g = 0$, respectively.

To find the corresponding variance of S_n, it is convenient to start from the well-known conditional variance formula (e.g., Ross 2019, ch. 3)

$$Var[S_n] = Var[E[S_n|D]] + E[Var[S_n|D]] \tag{2.54}$$

We just noticed that $E[S_n|D]$ equals $D \cdot a(n)$, and so the first summand on the right-hand side of Eq. (2.54) is given by

$$Var[D \cdot a(n)] = Var[D] \cdot [a(n)]^2 = 4g(1 - g) [a(n)]^2$$

where $a(n)$ is given by Eq. (2.38).

As for the second summand on the right-hand side of Eq. (2.54), we know from Eq. (2.41) that $Var[S_n|D]$ is actually independent of the initial directional state, that is, independent of D. Therefore, the second summand on the right-hand side of Eq. (2.54) is simply equal to the variance result that we have obtained in Eq. (2.41) for the cases $g = 0$ and $g = 1$. Relative to the case of a fixed initial directional state, randomizing the initial directional state adds a further variance component which is equal to $4g(1 - g) [a(n)]^2$. Clearly, this added variance component is zero if the initial direction is fixed ($g = 0$ or $g = 1$). It is maximal, and equal to $[a(n)]^2$, if $g = \frac{1}{2}$ in which case the variance $Var[S_n]$ of the position after n steps will be equal to $c(n)$, as given by Eq. (2.41).

2.5 More General Random Walks

The simple random walk is characterized by two basic properties which may both be relaxed. First, transitions occur only to the two nearest neighbor states. Second, steps to the left and right neighbor state always have the same, fixed probabilities, p and $1 - p$, independent of the current position of the walk. Note that even for the correlated random walk discussed in Sect. 2.4, the step probabilities were allowed to depend on the direction of the previous step, but not on the current position of the walk. In this section, we describe two widely used elementary models which illustrate ways in which these assumptions may be relaxed.

2.5.1 The Ehrenfest Model

The Ehrenfest (1907; Kohlrausch and Schrödinger 1926) model is a classic example that relaxes the second of the assumptions just described while keeping the first. In the Ehrenfest model, transitions still occur only between neighbored states; however, the transition probabilities vary according to the present position.

Consider m balls numbered $1, \ldots, m$ and two urns which we will call the left and the right urn. Initially, there are r balls in the right urn and $m - r$ balls in the left urn. The basic rule for transitions is as follows: at any step, a number $1, \ldots, m$ is drawn at random (each number having probability $1/m$), and the ball with that number is transferred from the urn it is currently in to the other urn. For example, if a large majority of balls is currently, say, in the right urn, then it is quite likely that in the next step, a ball will be transferred from the right into the left urn. The main effect of this transition rule is to implement a restoring force toward the state in which there is the same number (i.e., $m/2$) of balls in both urns. Moreover, this force is stronger the further the current state of the urns is away from this equilibrium state.

Let us call the number of balls in the right urn the *state*, or *position*, of the process. Denote as $N(k)$ the state of the process after $k \geq 0$ steps and as $\mathsf{E}[N(k)]$ its mean position. The initial state is $N(0) = r$, where $0 \leq r \leq m$. The basic transition rule then means that if the present state is N, then the process moves in the next step either to state $N - 1$ or to state $N + 1$ and the probabilities of these transitions are N/m and $1 - N/m$, respectively.

At what position will this process on average be after $k + 1$ steps, assuming it started in state r? Conditioning on the position $N(k)$ after k steps, we get

$$\mathsf{E}[N(k+1)] = \mathsf{E}\{\mathsf{E}[N(k+1)|N(k)]\} =$$
$$\mathsf{E}\left\{ [N(k) - 1] \cdot \frac{N(k)}{m} + [N(k) + 1] \cdot \left(1 - \frac{N(k)}{m}\right) \right\} \qquad (2.55)$$

because conditional on $N(k)$ the process moves with probability $N(k)/m$ down to position $N(k) - 1$ and with probability $1 - N(k)/m$ up to position $N(k) + 1$. Simplifying in Eq. (2.55) the bracketed expression within the expectation, we get a first-order difference equation in k

$$E[N(k+1)] = 1 + \left(1 - \frac{2}{m}\right) E[N(k)] \tag{2.56}$$

The solution of Eq. (2.56) satisfying the initial condition $E[N(0)] = r$ is

$$E[N(k)] = \frac{m}{2} + \left(r - \frac{m}{2}\right)\left(1 - \frac{2}{m}\right)^k \tag{2.57}$$

Equation (2.57) shows that on average, the process tends to the balanced state $m/2$, independent of the starting state r. Moreover, the approach to this limit will take more time (steps) the more extreme the starting state r is, and the larger the number m of balls. The cases $m = 1$ and $m = 2$ are quite instructive. For $m = 1$, the process oscillates deterministically between the states 0 and 1, in accordance with Eq. (2.57). For $m = 2$, there are only three states, 0, 1, and 2. From the boundary states 0 and 2, the process necessarily moves back to position 1; conversely, from state 1, it moves with equal probability to 0 and 2. This implies that for all $k > 0$, we must have $E[N(k)] = 1$, as Eq. (2.57) states.

In the basic Ehrenfest model, the process goes on indefinitely, as there are no absorbing states. However, we may still ask, as we did for simple random walks, how long it takes on average for the process to reach certain states for the first time.

To this end, denote as $Q_m(i)$, $i = 0, 1, \ldots, m - 1$ the mean first-passage time from state i to $i + 1$. Clearly, from these quantities, the mean first-passage time from any state to any other state is easily computed. For example, the first-passage time from state i to $i + 2$ is the sum of the first-passage time from state i to $i + 1$, plus the first-passage time from state $i + 1$ to $i + 2$. Similarly, for reasons of symmetry, the mean first-passage time from state i down to $i - 1$ must be equal to the mean first-passage time from state $m - i$ up to $m - i + 1$.

Consider, then, first passages from state i to $i + 1$. Either the process moves immediately in the first step from state i up to state $i + 1$; this case has probability $1 - i/m$, and if it occurs, then the first passage took just 1 step. Or, the process first moves from state i down to state $i - 1$, which has probability i/m. In this case, i.) one step is consumed, ii.) the process must first get from state $i - 1$ back to state i, and iii.) it must then get from state i to state $i + 1$. The duration of the whole first passage from i to $i + 1$ is in this case the sum of all three components involved, and so its average is $1 + Q_m(i - 1) + Q_m(i)$. This gives

$$Q_m(i) = 1 \cdot \left(1 - \frac{i}{m}\right) + [1 + Q_m(i - 1) + Q_m(i)] \cdot \frac{i}{m}$$

$$= \frac{m}{m - i} + \frac{i}{m - i} \cdot Q_m(i - 1) \tag{2.58}$$

Evidently, if all balls are in the left urn (state $i = 0$), then the next step must lead to one ball being transferred to the right urn, which means that for $i = 0$, the condition $Q_m(0) = 1$ must hold. Thus, we can in principle use the recursive relation Eq. (2.58) to compute $Q_m(i)$ successively for all $i = 1, \ldots, m - 1$ and from the $Q_m(i)$ in turn the mean first-passage times between any two states. An explicit solution of Eq. (2.58) is

$$Q_m(i) = \frac{1}{\binom{m-1}{i}} \sum_{k=0}^{i} \binom{m}{k} \tag{2.59}$$

As pointed out above, based on the $Q_m(i)$, we may now compute the mean first-passage time from any state to any other state. Figure 2.14 shows as a case of special interest the mean first-passage time from the balanced start state $r = m/2$ to the extreme state (m) in which all balls are in the right urn. The ordinate is logarithmic, and so the nearly linear increase of the function shown in Fig. 2.14 for medium and large m indicates that the mean first-passage time tends to increase exponentially in m.

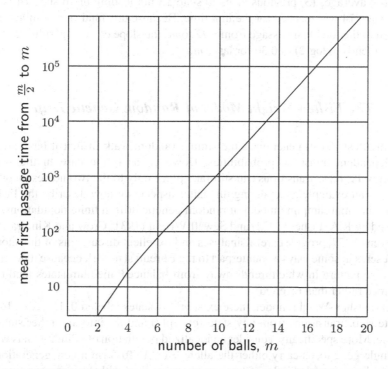

Fig. 2.14 Mean number of steps (ordinate) in the Ehrenfest model until all balls are for the first time contained in the right urn, shown here as a function of the number m of balls (abscissa). At the start, both urns contain $r = m/2$ balls. For example, starting with $r = 7$ balls in each urn, it takes on average nearly 18,000 steps until all $m = 14$ balls are for the first time collected in the right urn. Note the logarithmic scale of the ordinate

As is clear from the basic dynamics of the model, this is in marked contrast to first passages into the other direction, from state m down to state $m/2$. To illustrate, starting with 7 balls in each urn, it takes on average 17 943 steps until all 14 balls are for the first time collected in the right urn. In contrast, the first passage into the other direction, from 14 balls all in the right urn to 7 balls in both urns takes on average less than just 14 steps!

Another aspect behind Fig. 2.14 characteristic of the dynamics underlying the Ehrenfest model is that the quantities $Q_m(i)$ in Eq. (2.59) increase sharply with i. That is, from states i that are already far away from the balanced state $m/2$, it becomes progressively harder to reach the next even less balanced state, $i + 1$.

As an extreme case, consider Eq. (2.59) for the case of $i = m - 1$. Using the identity $\sum_{k=0}^{m} \binom{m}{k} = 2^m$, we note that for the final transition from state $m - 1$ to m on average, $Q_m(m - 1) = 2^m - 1$ steps are required. For example, in the case $m = 14$ just considered, it takes on average 17 943 steps to get for the first time from the balanced state $m/2 = 7$ to the extreme state $m = 14$. By far, the dominant portion of this overall duration is contributed by the final mean first-passage time from first reaching state 13 on to state 14, which alone requires on average 16 383 steps. This means that the total trip from state 7 to state 14 typically consists of many (on average, 13) previous visits to state 13 not leading on to state 14 before finally state 14 was reached for the first time. Because this final step dominates the duration of the total first passage from $m/2$ to m, the slope of the logarithmic plot in Fig. 2.14 tends to $\log(2) \approx 0.30$ for large m.

2.5.2   The Fisher–Wright Model of Random Genetic Drift

The Ehrenfest model generalizes the simple random walk in that it has variable, state-dependent transition probabilities. However, as is the case in the simple random walk, these transitions can still take place only to the two nearest neighbor states. As an example generalizing this latter aspect, we now describe the Fisher–Wright binomial sampling model of random genetic drift in finite populations, first proposed by R.A. Fisher (1922) and Sewall Wright (1931; Crow and Kimura 1970, and Ewens 1977, provide careful analyses and excellent discussions of this model). It represents in some ways a counterpart to the Ehrenfest model, because it describes a dynamic pattern in which trends away from balanced, medium states tend to be reinforced rather than reverted.

In the Fisher–Wright model, there exist $m + 1$ states labeled $0, 1, \ldots, m$. In any discrete step, transitions from any state (except 0 and m) into any other state are possible. More specifically, consider an idealized population of m individuals which at a single gene locus carry either the allele a or A. To form a new generation, m individuals are sampled independently, one-by-one and with replacement, from the current generation. The allele (a or A) of the selected individual is copied for one future individual. After m future individuals have been formed in this way, together they represent the new generation, the old generation being discarded. Note that any specific individual in the current generation may be selected exactly one time, or several times, or even never, much like the number of offspring per individual in real-world populations varies.[1]

One way to think about this process is as successive *binomial urns*, representing the successive generations. Suppose in the urn (generation) number n there are i allele-a individuals. If an individual from generation n is selected, its allele is copied to one future individual that is placed into a new, separate urn which forms the generation $n + 1$. The selected individual is placed back into its generation n urn, and the process stops when the urn for generation $n + 1$ contains m individuals. For any random selection of an individual from generation n, the probability is i/m that the selected allele (and thus that of the corresponding descendant in generation $n+1$) is a. From the assumption of independent draws with replacement, the probability to obtain j allele-a individuals in generation $n + 1$, given there were i of them in generation n, is then equal to the binomial

$$ p_{ij} = \binom{m}{j} \left(\frac{i}{m} \right)^{j} \left(1 - \frac{i}{m} \right)^{m-j} \tag{2.60} $$

In effect, Eq. (2.60) defines the probabilities in the Fisher–Wright model for one-step transitions of the present state i into the state j.

How many allele-a individuals will there on average be in generation k when in the initial generation ($k = 0$) there were r of them? To address this question, define the state $N(k)$ to be the number N of individuals in generation k carrying the a-allele. To relate successive generations, we condition on the value of $N(k)$. Given $N(k)$, the conditional expectation of $N(k + 1)$ is given by the mean of the corresponding binomial distribution, with parameters m and $N(k)/m$, that is, by $N(k)$. In terms of conditional expectation, we may write this relation more succinctly as $\mathsf{E}[N(k + 1)|N(k)] = N(k)$. Simply, if $N(k)$ individuals of the present generation carry the a-allele, then on average the same number will carry it in the next generation, too. More formally,

$$ \mathsf{E}[N(k + 1)] = \mathsf{E}\{ \mathsf{E}[N(k + 1)|N(k)] \} = \mathsf{E}[N(k)] \tag{2.61} $$

because $\mathsf{E}[N(k + 1)|N(k)] = N(k)$. As $E[N(0)] = r$, by induction, the same is true for any k.

One approach to find the corresponding variance of $N(k)$ is to use the conditional variance formula Eq. (2.54). Conditioning on the value of $N(k)$, we may apply this

---

[1] Many standard models in genetics assume per individual and gene segment two alleles, so that the allele combination of each individual at the segment considered is AA, Aa, or aa. In these models, one allele per individual is selected at random and paired with another randomly selected allele from a second individual, producing again one of the combinations AA, Aa, or aa. As long as we are only interested in the overall frequency of A and a (and not in the relative proportions of AA, Aa, and aa), the binomial sampling model is conceptually simpler.

equation to get information about $\text{Var}[N(k+1)]$, in the form

$$\text{Var}[N(k+1)] = \text{Var}[\text{E}[N(k+1)|N(k)]] + \text{E}[\text{Var}[N(k+1)|N(k)]] \quad (2.62)$$

We already know that given $N(k)$ the conditional expectation $\text{E}[N(k+1)|N(k)] = N(k)$. Similarly, given $N(k)$, the variance of $N(k+1)$ in the Fisher–Wright model is given by the binomial variance $m\,[N(k)/m]\,[1 - N(k)/m]$. Inserting these facts into Eq. (2.62) and using our previous result $\text{E}[N(k)] = r$, we get

$$\text{Var}[N(k+1)] = \text{Var}[N(k)] + \text{E}\left[m\,\frac{N(k)}{m}\left(1 - \frac{N(k)}{m}\right)\right]$$

$$= \text{Var}[N(k)] + r - \frac{1}{m}\,\text{E}[N^2(k)] \quad (2.63)$$

Applying the relation $\text{Var}[N(k)] = \text{E}[N^2(k)] - \text{E}^2[N(k)]$, we see that Eq. (2.63) represents a first-order difference equation for $\text{Var}[N(k)]$ in the generational variable k which is readily solved. The solution for $k \geq 0$ is

$$\text{Var}[N(k)] = r(m - r)\left[1 - \left(1 - \frac{1}{m}\right)^k\right] \quad (2.64)$$

Clearly, for the starting generation ($k = 0$), the initial number r of allele$-a$ individuals is fixed, and thus the variance of $N(0)$ is zero. According to Eq. (2.64), the variance of the number of allele$-a$ individuals increases from generation to generation until it finally converges to the limit of $r(m - r)$.

The transition probabilities in Eq. (2.60) mean that in every step, there is a nonzero probability to get into state 0 or state m. Given the basic mechanism, both of these states are absorbing. For example, if all m individuals in one generation carry the allele a, then A has died away, and all generations following it will also be purely a. In genetic theory, the event of entering these absorbing states is called *fixation*: once entered, these states are never left again. As illustrated in Fig. 2.15, the Fisher–Wright model thus describes an inherent tendency to extremes according to which the state variance around a constant mean of r is ever increasing (cf., Eq. (2.64)). If the process of generational reproduction goes on forever, it will eventually (with probability 1) end up either in state 0 or in state m. This raises the question of how likely it is for a population to end up in state 0 vs. in state m, considered as a function of both, the starting state, r, and the population size, m.

Based on our previous result about $\text{E}[N(k)] = r$, it is not difficult to answer this question. In the limit as $k \to \infty$, either none or all of the m individuals forming one generation will carry the allele a. Let us denote as $Q_m(r)$ the probability of the latter event, that is, of ultimate fixation in state m, where r is the starting state and m the (constant) size of the population. Now, we have seen from Eq. (2.61) that the mean state for any generation k is equal to r, and so, weighting states by their

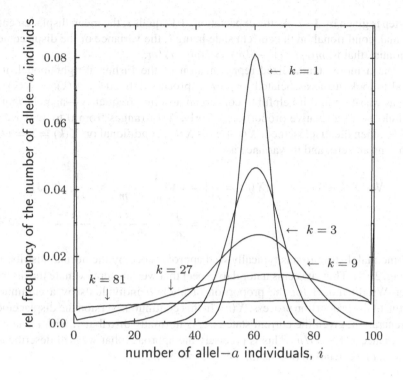

Fig. 2.15 Relative frequency (ordinate) of the number of allele−a individuals (abscissa) in a small population of $m = 100$ after $k = 1, 9, 27, 81$ generations; the start state is $r = 60$. For more clarity, the discrete probabilities per distribution are joined by lines. In the first generation, $k = 1$, the distribution is binomial, with parameters $m = 100$ and $\frac{r}{m} = 0.6$. In later generations, the frequencies cumulate at the two absorbing states $i = 0$ and $i = 100$. Ultimately, the distribution is concentrated at these two values, with probabilities of $1 - \frac{r}{m} = 0.4$ (for $i = 0$) and $\frac{r}{m} = 0.6$ (for $i = 100$). For all generations, the mean number of allele−a individuals remains constant at $r = 60$

probabilities, we must have that

$$m \cdot Q_m(r) + 0 \cdot [1 - Q_m(r)] = r \tag{2.65}$$

which means that $Q_m(r) = \frac{r}{m}$. Thus, we can interpret the limiting variance $r(m-r)$ in Eq. (2.64) for large k as resulting from a mixture of the two fixation states in which either all (probability r/m) or none (probability $1 - r/m$) of the m individuals carry the allele a.

A natural question to ask is how long on average it takes until fixation occurs? Although straightforward in principle, we will see in Sect. 6.2.3 that this question is much easier answered for a continuous version of the Fisher–Wright model. To prepare ideas leading to this version, consider that given the process is currently in state i, its (random) state **J** in the next generation is a binomial random variable with parameters m and i/m and thus mean i. Clearly, the *displacement* occurring in the next step is given by $\mathbf{J} - i$. As the expectation of $\mathbf{J}$ equals i, the mean displacement is zero, and, conditional on the current state being i, the variance of the displacement is binomial, that is, $m(i/m)(1 - i/m) = i(m - i)/m$.

To get a more standardized representation of the Fisher–Wright model, it is natural to look at the associated *proportion* process defined by $X(k) = N(k)/m$, much as we often find it helpful to convert an absolute frequency—namely, that of the allele a—to a relative proportion. Clearly, $X(k)$ ranges from 0 to 1. If we let $x = i/m$, then the displacement $X(k + 1) - X(k)$, conditional on $X(k) = x = i/m$, still has mean zero, and its variance is

$$\text{Var}[X(k + 1) - X(k)|X(k) = \frac{i}{m}] = \text{Var}[\frac{\mathbf{J}}{m} - \frac{i}{m}] = \frac{1}{m^2} \text{Var}[\mathbf{J}]$$

$$= \frac{1}{m^2} \frac{i(m - i)}{m} = \frac{x(1 - x)}{m} \qquad (2.66)$$

The binomial distribution is typically well approximated by the normal distribution (cf., Fig. 2.15). Thus, it seems natural to expect that we can approximate the discrete Fisher–Wright model for the proportion of allele-a individuals by a continuous version, of the proportion process, $X(k)$. In this continuous version the displacement per generation, given the current state is x, is normally distributed with mean zero and variance $x(1 - x)/m$. This is precisely the approach that we will describe and pursue in more detail in Sects. 5.3.2, 6.2.3, and 6.3.5.

2.6   Exercises

1. Derive the limit of $p \to \frac{1}{2}$ for the expected first-passage time given by Eq. (2.21) and also for the conditional expected first-passage time in Eq. (2.26). Then confirm, using Eq. (2.14), that for $p = \frac{1}{2}$, the expected first-passage time is a weighted mean of the two conditional expected first-passage times.

2. In a population of consumers, a fraction of p favors brand A over B. Consumers are randomly sampled one after another from this population and have to make a forced choice to indicate their preference either for A or for B. The investigator stops sampling new consumers when the difference between pro-A choices and pro-B choices reaches for the first time a critical value of $+a$ or $-a$. In the first case, the investigator concludes that a majority of consumers prefers A and in the second that a majority prefers B. For given numbers a and p, how likely is it that the study reaches a correct conclusion? How many consumers will on average be sampled? The investigator can only influence a, not p. What is in your view a reasonable choice of a, and in which way is this value influenced by p?

3. In certain sports (e.g., traditional tiebreak rules in tennis or table tennis), two players A and B compete for points until one of them achieves a lead of 2 points. Assume that player A wins each point with probability p and that successive rounds are independent.

How likely is it that player A will win? How many rounds are on average required until a winner is found? What is the average number of rounds given that player A wins? What changes if the required lead is three (or a) points rather than two?

4. From the definition of a pgf given in Eq. (2.29), for any non-defective (regular) distribution of a positive random variable N, we must have $g(1) = 1$. On the other hand, for a defective distribution we have $g(1) = r < 1$, where $r = \sum_{n=1}^{\infty} P(N = n)$. For example, for a simple random walk, we know from Eq. (2.9) that for the distribution of the number of steps to reach the barrier at $a = 1$, the constant $r = p/(1 - p)$ when $p < \frac{1}{2}$.

Further, for a defective distribution, the expression

$$\frac{g'(1)}{g(1)} = \frac{\sum_{n=1}^{\infty} n \cdot P(N = n)}{\sum_{n=1}^{\infty} P(N = n)}$$

represents a weighted mean that can be interpreted as the conditional mean, given that the random variable N takes a finite value. Note that this more general definition contains regular distributions (when $r = 1$) as a special case.

Recall that $\sqrt{a^2} = |a|$ for all real a; for example, $\sqrt{(-3)^2} = +3$. With this fact in mind, show from Eq. (2.31) that for $p < \frac{1}{2}$, the value of $g(1) = p/(1 - p)$, whereas for $p > \frac{1}{2}$, we have $g(1) = 1$; see Fig. 2.5.

Also show that for $p < \frac{1}{2}$, we have $g'(1) = p/[(1 - p)(1 - 2p)]$, whereas for $p > \frac{1}{2}$, we have $g'(1) = 1/(2p - 1)$. Use these facts and Eq. (2.31) to confirm the finding in Eq. (2.18) that for $p > \frac{1}{2}$, the mean number of steps to reach the barrier at $a > 0$ is equal to $a/(2p - 1) = a/\mu$. Also conclude that for $p < \frac{1}{2}$, the conditional mean number of steps to reach the barrier at $a > 0$, given it is reached at all, is equal to $a/(1 - 2p) = a/|\mu|$.

5. (a) For paths with unit steps such as shown in Fig. 2.16, argue much as we did to obtain Eq. (2.7) that the total number N of paths leading from $(0|\alpha)$ to $(x|\beta)$ is given by ($\alpha > 0$, $\beta \geq 0$)

$$N = \binom{p + q}{p} = \binom{x}{\frac{1}{2}(x + \beta - \alpha)} \tag{$*$}$$

where p is the number of upward steps and q the number of downward steps, so that $p + q$ is the total number x of steps and $p - q$ is the overall vertical displacement $\beta - \alpha$ during these x steps. For $(*)$ to hold, we must have that $x \geq |\alpha - \beta|$ and that x and $|\alpha - \beta|$ have the same parity.

Observe that some of the N paths, like the one labeled (i) in Fig. 2.16, never reach the horizontal axis (the line $y = 0$), whereas all other paths, like the one labeled (ii) in Fig. 2.16, do reach the line $y = 0$ at least once. Denote as N_+ the number of the former paths and as N_- the number of the latter paths; clearly, $N = N_+ + N_-$.

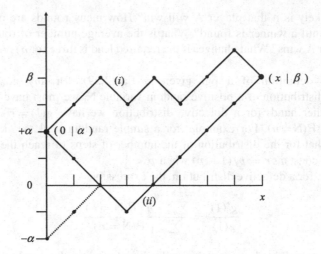

Fig. 2.16 Two paths leading from $(0|\alpha)$ to $(x|\beta)$, illustrated here for $x = 8$, $\alpha = 2$, and $\beta = 4$, so that $p = 5$ steps must be upward and $q = 3$ steps downward. There are in all $N = 56$ paths leading from $(0|2)$ to $(8|4)$. The path labeled (i) is one of $N_+ = 48$ which lead to $(x|\beta)$ without ever reaching the line $y = 0$. The path labeled (ii) is one of $N_- = 8$ which lead to $(x|\beta)$ after first reaching the line $y = 0$. The dotted path starting from $(0| - \alpha)$ is the mirror image of path (ii) until both first reach the line $y = 0$. Note that any path from $(0| - \alpha)$ to $(x|\beta)$ necessarily must reach the line $y = 0$ at least once

(b) Based on the dotted mirror path shown in Fig. 2.16, explain why the number N_- of paths leading from $(0|\alpha)$ to $(x|\beta)$ which at least once reach the line $y = 0$ is the same as the number of paths (of any sort) leading from $(0| - \alpha)$ to $(x|\beta)$, an argument sometimes called the reflection principle. According to similar considerations as in (a), this latter number is

$$N_- = \binom{p' + q'}{p'} = \binom{x}{\frac{1}{2}(x + \beta + \alpha)} \tag{**}$$

Here, p' is the number of upward steps, and q' the number of downward steps of the path from $(0| - \alpha)$ to $(x|\beta)$, so that $p' + q'$ is again the total number x of steps and $p' - q'$ is the overall vertical displacement $\beta + \alpha$ during these x steps.

(c) Conclude from (*) and (**) that the number N_+ of paths starting at $(0|\alpha)$ and ending at $(x|\beta)$ which never reach the line $y = 0$ is

$$N_+ = N - N_- = \binom{x}{\frac{1}{2}(x + \beta - \alpha)} - \binom{x}{\frac{1}{2}(x + \beta + \alpha)} \tag{***}$$

(d) Conclude further from (***) that the number of paths from $(0|\alpha)$ to $(x|0)$ which reach the line $y = 0$ for the first time with their final step is for $x \geq \alpha$ equal to

$$\frac{\alpha}{x} \binom{x}{\frac{1}{2}(x + \alpha)} \qquad (****)$$

Observe that all of these paths must necessarily pass through $(x - 1|1)$ without ever reaching the line $y = 0$ before, which corresponds to (***) with $x - 1$ steps and $\beta = 1$, and then in their final step move from $(x - 1|1)$ to $(x|0)$.

Conclude that among all paths which start at $(0|\alpha)$ and end at $(x|0)$, the relative proportion (probability) of paths which at $(x|0)$ reach the line $y = 0$ for the first time is equal to α/x (cf., the case $\alpha = x$). Argue that by symmetry of all paths starting at $(0|0)$ and ending at $(x|\alpha)$, a fraction of α/x reaches the line $y = \alpha$ for the first time with the last step.

6. Consider a symmetric simple random walk starting at 0 when $a > 0$ is an absorbing barrier. Let $p_a(i, n)$ represent the probability that after n steps, the walk occupies position $i \leq a$. Explain why the relations

$$p_a(i, n) = \frac{1}{2} \left[p_a(i + 1, n - 1) + p_a(i - 1, n - 1) \right]$$

hold for all states $i < a - 1$. In effect, these relations correspond to the forward Eq. (2.3) for the unrestricted evolution and show that the "local" dynamics for states distant from the barrier a is just as for a random walk without barriers. In contrast, the state $a - 1$ can only be reached from $a - 2$ which means that

$$p_a(a - 1, n) = \frac{1}{2} p_a(a - 2, n - 1)$$

Finally, the state a is absorbing so that

$$p_a(a, n) = p_a(a, n - 1) + \frac{1}{2} p_a(a - 1, n - 1)$$

Use Eq. (***) of Exercise 5 to show that

$$p_a(i, n) = 2^{-n} \cdot \left[\binom{n}{\frac{n-i}{2}} - \binom{n}{a + \frac{n-i}{2}} \right]$$

where the binomial coefficient $\binom{b}{c} = 0$ when $c < 0$ or $c > b$.

Note that for a given value of n summing $p_a(i, n)$ across all states $i < a$ represents the total probability for the walk *not* to be absorbed after n steps; we thus have the basic relation

$$1 - p_a(a, n) = \sum_{i=-\infty}^{a-1} p_a(i, n)$$

(evidently, the lowest contributing index $i = -n$).

7. For the case of the symmetric simple random walk, Eq. (2.7) implies that

$$p(\Delta, n) = \binom{n}{\frac{n}{2} + \frac{\Delta}{2}} \left(\frac{1}{2}\right)^n$$

where n is the number of steps and $\Delta = m - k$ is the net displacement of the walk during these n steps. Use Stirling's approximation (e.g., Feller 1968, ch. 2)

$$\binom{2m}{m + r} \approx \frac{1}{\sqrt{m\pi}} \exp\left(-\frac{r^2}{m}\right) 2^{2m}$$

to show that for large n, the expression $p(\Delta, n)$ tends to the continuous limit

$$p^*(\Delta, n) = 2 \cdot \frac{1}{\sqrt{2\pi n}} \exp\left(-\frac{\Delta^2}{2n}\right)$$

that is, to a normal distribution with mean zero and variance n, multiplied by a factor of 2.

Explain the factor of 2 by considering that for a walk with, say, $n = 100$ steps, Δ varies from -100 to $+100$ in steps of size 2; odd values of Δ are impossible. For example, to approximate $p(\Delta = 0, n)$ by the continuous limit, we need to consider the area under the normal density with mean zero and variance n between -1 and $+1$ (an interval of width 2), which is roughly equal to $p^*(0, n)$. Similarly, for the next possible value $\Delta = 2$, the expression $p(2, n)$ would be approximated by the area under the normal density with mean zero and variance n between $+1$ and $+3$, which is roughly equal to $p^*(2, n)$.

Chapter 3
Small Steps at High Speed: The Diffusion Limit

3.1 Small Steps at High Speed: The Diffusion Limit

In Chap. 2, we studied simple random walks which in each time unit move one spatial unit to the left or right. After a sufficiently long time, the position of the walk will then represent the sum of a large number of component steps which individually are small relative to the spatial scale of the walk at large. According to the central limit theorem, the sum of identical and independent components will under rather weak conditions tend to the normal distribution. Consider the position $X(t)$ that a freely evolving random walk occupies across many independent realizations at a fixed time t which is large relative to the duration of a single step (i.e., after a large number of steps). It is then natural to expect that the relative frequencies of the various positions $X(t)$ may be well approximated by a normal distribution.

In this chapter, we describe some main concepts that help in understanding heuristically how, and under which conditions, processes which are generically discrete in time and space may eventually tend to diffusion processes which are continuous in time and space. This continuous framework will permit us to cover processes that are more general than the simple random walk. In many cases, the continuous treatment leads more easily and more directly to information about major characteristics of the specific process in question. This is partly because the continuous treatment does not rely on individual (albeit often ingenious) case-by-case arguments used for some of the discrete models that we considered in Chap. 2. Rather, the continuous framework relies on a more uniform approach that exploits standard mathematical tools such as differential equations, which help to streamline the process of investigating practically relevant properties of standard diffusion processes. To arrive at this more versatile continuous framework, we first need to reconsider the simple random walk in a slightly more general setup.

In this more general scenario, let us assume that each step of the walk has size $+\Delta x$ or $-\Delta x$ and that the duration of any step is Δt. Our strategic aim is to look at conditions under which the joint limit of $\Delta t \to 0$ and $\Delta x \to 0$ leads to a meaningful

© Springer Nature Switzerland AG 2022
W. Schwarz, *Random Walk and Diffusion Models*,
https://doi.org/10.1007/978-3-031-12100-5_3

continuous diffusion process $\{X(t), t \geq 0\}$ where $X(t)$ is the position of the process at time t. For example, $X(t)$ must for any t have a well-defined density function f which for $t = 0$ is concentrated at the start point x_0, just as a simple random walk occupies with probability 1 its starting point. To introduce and emphasize some main conceptual points, the present chapter considers the symmetric simple random walk without drift, that is, the case of $p = \frac{1}{2}$. The next chapter then looks in considerable detail at the modifications needed when $p \neq \frac{1}{2}$, and the chapters following it look at still more general cases.

Assume that t denotes the moment at which exactly n steps are completed, that is, $t = n\Delta t$. We consider t as a fixed quantity and imagine a limiting process in which the step duration Δt decreases toward zero and the number n of steps increases, so that their product $t = n \cdot \Delta t$ remains fixed.

The position $X(\Delta t)$ after the first step is, with equal probability, $+\Delta x$ or $-\Delta x$. Therefore, we have

$$\mathsf{E}[X(\Delta t)] = 0 \quad \text{and} \quad \mathsf{Var}[X(\Delta t)] = \mathsf{E}[X^2(\Delta t)] = (\Delta x)^2$$

Clearly, $X(t = n\Delta t)$ is the sum of n independent similar steps; therefore, the mean

$$\mathsf{E}[X(t)] = n \cdot \mathsf{E}[X(\Delta t)] = 0 \tag{3.1}$$

and the variance of the individual displacements are additive:

$$\mathsf{Var}[X(t)] = n \cdot \mathsf{Var}[X(\Delta t)] = n \cdot (\Delta x)^2$$

$$= \frac{t}{\Delta t} \cdot (\Delta x)^2 = \frac{(\Delta x)^2}{\Delta t} \cdot t \tag{3.2}$$

For finite values of Δx and Δt, the variable $X(t = n\Delta t)$ has a symmetric binomial distribution over the $n + 1$ possible discrete positions, separated by $2\Delta x$, from $x = -n\Delta x$ to $x = +n\Delta x$, with the expected value 0 as its most probable position. For example, after $n = 2$ steps, the process can only be at positions $-2\Delta x$, 0, or $+2\Delta x$, with probabilities of $\frac{1}{4}$, $\frac{1}{2}$, and $\frac{1}{4}$, respectively.

To obtain a meaningful limit, Eq. (3.2) suggests to let $\Delta t \to 0$ and $\Delta x \to 0$ in a way such that the quantity $(\Delta x)^2/\Delta t$ converges to a finite limit. We will write this limit as

$$\lim_{\Delta t \to 0, \Delta x \to 0} \frac{(\Delta x)^2}{\Delta t} = \sigma^2 > 0 \tag{3.3}$$

which essentially means that Δx and Δt individually tend to zero in a way so that $\Delta x = \sigma\sqrt{\Delta t}$. This implies that for small values—such as we are considering here—the step size Δx is typically much *larger* than the step duration Δt (note that, e.g., $\sqrt{0.01} = 0.1$).

What interpretation can be given to the limit σ^2 appearing in Eq. (3.3)? Note that each time step has duration Δt and the displacement is $\pm \Delta x = \pm \sigma \sqrt{\Delta t}$, which means that the squared displacement will be $\sigma^2 \Delta t$. Given that in the symmetric random walk the mean displacement per step is zero, $\sigma^2 \Delta t$ is equal to the variance of the displacement per Δt. Therefore, as already suggested by the choice of the symbol, σ^2 is the variance of the displacement per time unit.

3.2 The Diffusion Equation

3.2.1 From Difference Equations to Differential Equations

In the following, we will often need the notion of the derivative of a function as the limit of the difference quotient (e.g., Stewart 2012, ch. 2). Recall that the difference quotient of a differentiable function f at x is defined as

$$\frac{f(x + \Delta x) - f(x)}{\Delta x} \tag{3.4}$$

In the limit of $\Delta x \to 0$, this expression defines the derivative of f at x, written as $f'(x)$, so that for small Δx, the difference quotient will be close to $f'(x)$.

Analogously, the second-order difference quotient is the difference quotient of f'. As $\Delta x \to 0$, we have

$$f''(x) \approx \frac{f(x + \Delta x) - 2f(x) + f(x - \Delta x)}{(\Delta x)^2} \tag{3.5}$$

An important aspect is that Eq. (3.4) may be interpreted as a numerical recipe of how a difference like $f(x + \Delta x) - f(x)$ can be approximated, namely, as $f'(x)\,\Delta x$. Similarly, Eq. (3.5) means that $f(x + \Delta x) - 2f(x) + f(x - \Delta x)$ is approximately equal to $(\Delta x)^2 f''(x)$. The error of these approximations will be small for small Δx and tend to zero as Δx tends to zero. In a sense, the distinction between difference quotients and derivatives is the formal analogy to the distinction between discrete random walks and continuous diffusion processes. It is therefore important to have a clear understanding that (under the usual regularity conditions) difference quotients are approximated by the corresponding derivatives when the Δ involved is small and converge to them when the Δ tends to zero. In the following, we will make use of this relation extensively.

With this background, we now consider a symmetric random walk and let $f(x, t)$ represent the probability to be at position x at time t. Clearly, this probability must also depend on the starting point x_0, but to focus on the actually varying quantities that are central to the derivation, we suppress x_0 for now and will add it later to a more complete notation. We again use the logic leading to the forward Eq. (2.3) and consider that for the walk to be at a fixed position $x = k\Delta x$ at time $(n + 1)\Delta t$, then at time $t = n\Delta t$ (i.e., one step before), the walk must have occupied either position $x = (k - 1)\Delta x$ or position $x = (k + 1)\Delta x$. In the first case, a step of $+\Delta x$ must have followed and in the second a step of size $-\Delta x$; both scenarios have probability $\frac{1}{2}$. As there are no other ways to arrive at $x = k\Delta x$ at time $(n + 1)\Delta t$, we get for the transition probability f the partial difference equation

$$f(k\Delta x, (n + 1)\Delta t) = \frac{1}{2} \cdot [f((k - 1)\Delta x, n\Delta t) + f((k + 1)\Delta x, n\Delta t)] \qquad (3.6)$$

As before regarding the variable t, we consider $x = k\Delta x$ as a fixed quantity and contemplate a limiting process with an increasing number, k, of steps of decreasing size, Δx. More specifically, we assume that the step size Δx decreases to zero, while k increases in a way such that the product $x = k\Delta x$ remains constant.

We next relate the partial difference Eq. (3.6) for f to difference quotients, as follows. First, we subtract $f(k\Delta x, n\Delta t)$ on both sides of Eq. (3.6) and divide through by Δt. The left-hand side of Eq. (3.6) then becomes

$$\frac{f(k\Delta x, (n + 1)\Delta t) - f(k\Delta x, n\Delta t)}{\Delta t}$$

which for fixed $x = k\Delta x, t = n\Delta t$, and $\Delta t \to 0$ tends to the partial derivative of f with respect to t.

Turning to the right-hand side of Eq. (3.6), we obtain after subtracting $f(k\Delta x, n\Delta t)$ and dividing by Δt

$$\frac{1}{2\Delta t} \cdot [f((k - 1)\Delta x, n\Delta t) - 2f(k\Delta x, n\Delta t) + f((k + 1)\Delta x, n\Delta t)]$$

which in view of Eq. (3.5) we rewrite in the equivalent form of

$$\frac{1}{2} \cdot \frac{(\Delta x)^2}{\Delta t} \cdot \frac{f((k - 1)\Delta x, n\Delta t) - 2f(k\Delta x, n\Delta t) + f((k + 1)\Delta x, n\Delta t)}{(\Delta x)^2}$$

As discussed above (see Eq. (3.3)), we consider the joint limit of Δx and Δt for which the first two factors of this expression tend to $\frac{1}{2}\sigma^2$. For fixed $t = n\Delta t$, the fraction forming the third factor is just equal to the second-order difference quotient of f with respect to x. According to Eq. (3.5), it thus converges for $\Delta x \to 0$ to the second derivative of f with respect to x, evaluated at the point $(k\Delta x, n\Delta t)$. Inserting the relations $t = n\Delta t$ and $x = k\Delta x$, we thus get from the partial difference Eq. (3.6) in the limit for f the partial differential equation

$$\frac{\partial f(x_0, x, t)}{\partial t} = \frac{1}{2}\sigma^2 \cdot \frac{\partial^2 f(x_0, x, t)}{\partial x^2} \qquad (3.7)$$

where we have added x_0 to the arguments of f to indicate, as mentioned above, that f must as well depend on x_0.

Equation (3.7) is called the forward equation for a simple diffusion process $\{X(t), t \geq 0\}$ with no systematic drift component. It relates changes of f in the time variable t to changes in the position (or state) variable x, for any given, fixed starting value x_0, and represents the continuous counterpart to the corresponding forward Eq. (2.3) for discrete simple random walks (in the symmetric case, $p = \frac{1}{2}$), as explained in Sect. 2.2.2.

Equation (3.7) is in itself not sufficient to specify the one particular solution f that we seek. For example, the functions $x_0 \exp(-\lambda t) \sin\left(x\frac{\sqrt{2\lambda}}{\sigma}\right)$ or $\exp\left(x_0 + \lambda t + x\frac{\sqrt{2\lambda}}{\sigma}\right)$ are for any λ solutions of Eq. (3.7). However, these solutions do not satisfy the initial condition at $t = 0$, which prescribes that at the start of the diffusion process, the entire probability mass must be concentrated at x_0. Fortunately, the probabilistic background of our derivation leads us directly to the unique appropriate solution of Eq. (3.7).

The limiting process considered above in effect appeals to the conditions under which the central limit theorem applies. In this idealized construction, the position of the process at any time t is the sum of a large number of independent and identically distributed random variables, representing the individual steps of the walk. Motivated by this background, we expect from the previous results Eqs. (3.1)– (3.3) that the solution of Eq. (3.7) will be a normal density, centered on its starting point x_0, and with variance $\sigma^2 t$. In fact, it is straightforward (if laborious) to verify that

$$f(x_0, x, t) = \frac{1}{\sigma\sqrt{2\pi t}} \cdot \exp\left[-\frac{(x - x_0)^2}{2\sigma^2 t}\right] \tag{3.8}$$

is for all x_0 a solution of Eq. (3.7).

Equation (3.8) means that for any t, the position variable $X(t)$ is normally distributed, centered on its starting point x_0, and with variance proportional to t. For small t, the density f is narrowly concentrated around its starting point x_0, but the variance of $X(t)$ increases in proportion to t, the factor of proportionality being σ^2, which explains the meaning of the limit indicated in Eq. (3.3).

By its construction based on the symmetric simple random walk, two important properties of the continuous limiting process characterized by Eq. (3.7) are that it has *independent increments* and that it inherits the Markovian property described for simple random walks in Sect. 2.1. The first property means that the displacements of the process in disjoint time intervals are independent. The continuous limiting process also has *stationary increments* which means that the distribution of the displacement in any time interval $[s, s + t]$ depends only on the length t of the interval, but not on when it starts, that is, not on s. This means that Eq. (3.8) also represents the density of the displacement of the process in any interval $[s, s + t]$ if we denote the starting point at time s as $X(s) = x_0$.

Note the different conceptual roles played by x and t in Eq. (3.8). That is, for any fixed t, the function f is a probability density in the spatial variable x. For example, the area under f for any fixed t is equal to 1. The values of x represent the possible values which the random variable $X(t)$ takes, whereas t is a deterministic parameter indexing time. For example, for a given, fixed x and varying t, we cannot, for example, interpret f as the density of the time needed to reach x.

Another important aspect of Eq. (3.8) is that we may write it as well in the form

$$f(x_0, x, t) = \frac{1}{\sigma\sqrt{2\pi t}} \cdot \exp\left[-\frac{(x_0 - x)^2}{2\sigma^2 t}\right]$$

which for reasons of symmetry shows that f will also satisfy the equation

$$\frac{\partial f(x_0, x, t)}{\partial t} = \frac{1}{2}\sigma^2 \cdot \frac{\partial^2 f(x_0, x, t)}{\partial x_0^2} \tag{3.9}$$

Equation (3.9) is called the backward equation for a simple diffusion process with no systematic drift component. It looks similar to the forward Eq. (3.7) but relates changes of f in the time variable t to changes in the starting variable x_0, for any given, fixed value of the position variable x. The backward Eq. (3.9) represents the continuous counterpart to the corresponding backward Eq. (2.4) for discrete simple random walks in the symmetric case, $p = \frac{1}{2}$, that was described in Sect. 2.2.2.

3.2.2 Fick's Laws, Galton's Board, and the Diffusion Equation

In Sect. 1.2.2, we have seen in some detail how two fairly plausible assumptions about the nature of physical diffusion processes made by A. Fick in 1855 lead to the simple diffusion equation (1.3) which is the same as the forward Eq. (3.7), with Fick's "diffusion constant" D replaced by $\frac{1}{2}\sigma^2$. It is instructive to relate the Fickian terminology of a "substance", thought of as a great number of diffusing particles (see Fig. 1.5), to a context in which the process of diffusion results as a limit of a simple random walk. To this end, we use the scheme of Galton's board to understand heuristically how to obtain Eq. (3.7) in much the same way in which we derived the forward diffusion equation from Fick's laws.

As shown in Fig. 1.3, the successive rows on Galton's board along the vertical dimension correspond to time t, and the horizontal displacement of the balls represent the x-coordinates. Let us assume it takes Δt for a ball to pass from one row to the next and that the wedges in any row are separated horizontally by Δx.

Consider the events on a Galton board at a position x in a small time interval $[t, t + \Delta t]$, which corresponds to the events when one "generation" of balls passes from one row to the next. To this end, let $F(x, t)$ be the proportion of balls to the left of x at time (row) t, that is, F is a (cumulative) distribution function with respect to x for any given t. Of course, F will also depend on the location x_0 of the funnel, corresponding to the starting point, but for now, we again suppress this quantity in our notation as it will remain fixed in the following.

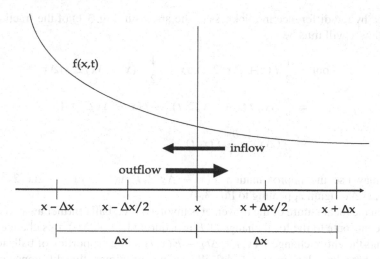

Fig. 3.1 At time t, the probability for a ball to be to the left of x is $F(x, t)$, and so the fraction contained in the small interval $[x - \Delta x, x]$ is given by $F(x, t) - F(x - \Delta x, t)$ which according to Eq. (3.4) we approximate by $f(x - \Delta x/2, t)\Delta x$. In a short time interval $[t, t + \Delta t]$, the change of $F(x, t)$ is governed by the local flows across the border at x. There will be an outflow from the left to the right across x equal to $\frac{1}{2} f(x - \Delta x/2, t)\Delta x$. At the same time, there will be an inflow from the right to the left across x equal to $\frac{1}{2} f(x + \Delta x/2, t)\Delta x$. Given the decrease of f at x, the outflow will be larger than the inflow, as indicated by the thickness of the arrows. The net change $F(x, t + \Delta t) - F(x, t)$ during the short time interval $[t, t + \Delta t]$ is the difference of the inflow minus the outflow. For small Δx, it tends to $\frac{1}{2} (\Delta x)^2 \frac{\partial f(x,t)}{\partial x}$.

Also, let $f(x, t)$ be the corresponding local density of balls at position x at time t, that is, $\frac{\partial F}{\partial x} = f(x, t)$. Thus, $F(x, t) - F(x - \Delta x, t)$ represents the proportion of all balls emanating at $t = 0$ from the funnel that will at time t be found in the small interval $[x - \Delta x, x]$. According to Eq. (3.4), we can approximate the difference $F(x, t) - F(x - \Delta x, t)$ by $f(x - \Delta x/2, t)\Delta x$, because $f(x, t)$ is the derivative of F with respect to x.

As indicated in Fig. 3.1, during the time interval $[t, t + \Delta t]$, half of the fraction of $f(x - \Delta x/2, t)\Delta x$ balls in the small interval $[x - \Delta x, x]$ will move one spatial step Δx to the right and thereby exit the region below x. The other half will move one spatial step Δx to the left and thus remain in the region below x. Similarly, at time t, a fraction of about $f(x + \Delta x/2, t)\Delta x$ balls will be found in the adjacent small interval $[x, x + \Delta x]$. Again, of these balls, one-half will move to the left, that is, enter the region below x from the right, whereas the other half will move to the right and thus remain in the region above x. The net change (inflow minus outflow,

indicated by the difference in thickness of the arrows in Fig. 3.1) of the fraction of
balls below x will thus be

$$in - out = \frac{1}{2} f(x + \Delta x/2, t)\Delta x - \frac{1}{2} f(x - \Delta x/2, t)\Delta x$$

$$= \frac{1}{2} \Delta x [f(x + \Delta x/2, t) - f(x - \Delta x/2, t)]$$

$$\approx \frac{1}{2} (\Delta x)^2 \frac{\partial}{\partial x} f(x, t)$$

as we may use the approximation $f(x + \Delta x/2, t)\Delta x - f(x - \Delta x/2, t) \approx \frac{\partial}{\partial x} f(x, t)\,\Delta x$, again appealing to Eq. (3.4).

Given the local nature of the movements involved (i.e., balls further away from x
cannot contribute to the local change of F at x during $[t, t + \Delta t]$), this change also
represents the entire change $F(x, t + \Delta t) - F(x, t)$ in the proportion of balls to the
left of x that takes place in $[t, t + \Delta t]$. We again approximate this difference in the
manner of Eq. (3.4) and obtain

$$F(x, t + \Delta t) - F(x, t) \approx \Delta t \frac{\partial}{\partial t} F(x, t) = \frac{1}{2} (\Delta x)^2 \frac{\partial}{\partial x} f(x, t) \quad (3.10)$$

Now, $F(x, t)$ is the distribution function giving the proportion of balls to the left of
x at time t. Therefore, its derivative with respect to x is the corresponding density
$f(x, t)$ at time t. Differentiating both sides of Eq. (3.10) with respect to x and
dividing by Δt give

$$\frac{\partial}{\partial t} f(x, t) = \frac{1}{2} \frac{(\Delta x)^2}{\Delta t} \frac{\partial^2}{\partial x^2} f(x, t)$$

Now going as before (Eq. (3.3)) to the limit $\Delta t \to 0$ and $\Delta x \to 0$ so that

$$\lim_{\Delta t \to 0, \Delta x \to 0} \frac{(\Delta x)^2}{\Delta t} = \sigma^2$$

we get the diffusion equation (3.7).

Recall that $F(x, t)$ is the proportion (probability) of balls below x at time
t. Dividing Eq. (3.10) by Δt gives the total change $F(x, t + \Delta t) - F(x, t)$ of
probability content in the interval below x per time unit in the interval $[t, t + \Delta t]$,
the net *flux* (flow, current) of probability across the coordinate x. As formulated, it
would be taken in the right-to-left direction because the expression is positive when
$F(x, t + \Delta t) > F(x, t)$, that is, when more balls are below x at time $t + \Delta t$ than
there were at time t. Dividing Eq. (3.10) by Δt, then again using Eq. (3.3), for small

steps and short durations, the limit is seen to be equal to

$$\frac{\partial}{\partial t} F(x, t) = \frac{1}{2} \sigma^2 \frac{\partial}{\partial x} f(x, t)$$

More conventionally, the flux is taken in the left-to-right (i.e., positive) direction, and so a negative sign must precede this expression, giving the standard left-to-right flux $J(x, t)$ at t across x as

$$J(x, t) = \frac{\partial}{\partial t} F(x, t) = -\frac{1}{2} \sigma^2 \frac{\partial}{\partial x} f(x, t) \qquad (3.11)$$

We can interpret Eq. (3.11) for the flux of probability across x as another form to express Fick's second assumption described in Sect. 1.2.2: in pure diffusion, the amount $J(x, t)$ of substance passing per time unit through a cross-section at x is proportional to the gradient of concentration at x, that is, proportional to $\frac{\partial}{\partial x} f(x, t)$. For example, in Fig. 3.1, f is decreasing at x so that $\frac{\partial}{\partial x} f(x, t)$ is negative and more mass is concentrated just to the left of x than just to the right of it. Therefore, from pure diffusion, we would then expect more probability mass to flow from left to right than vice versa, producing a positive left-to-right net flux across x.

We know that the appropriate particular solution to the forward diffusion equation is Eq. (3.8). In terms of Galton's board, the meaning of the initial condition satisfied by the solution $f(x_0, x, t)$ as $t \rightarrow 0$ is that initially all balls enter the board through the funnel that is centered on x_0. The variance parameter σ^2 in Eq. (3.8) corresponds to (twice) the diffusion coefficient D discussed in Sect. 1.2.2. In classical diffusion, D depends, for example, on the temperature of the solution. In relation to Galton's board, σ^2 controls the increase of spread of the balls per time unit as they run from row to row through the board. For example, if the vertical distance of the rows is reduced, then the balls will pass more rows per time unit, and the spread of the balls running through the board will increase faster.

3.3   An Alternative Derivation: The Moment-Generating Function

Equation (3.8) is a basic result, and so it is instructive to introduce and illustrate different techniques to arrive at it, as each of these techniques can be adapted to handle more complex cases. One such powerful technique in the context of random processes is the moment-generating function (for short mgf; Cox and Miller 1965, ch. 2.3, provide an excellent exposition), the counterpart to the pgf of discrete distributions, described in Sect. 2.3.6.

The mgf of the density of a random variable $\mathbf{X}$ is its two-sided Laplace transform, $m(\theta) = \mathsf{E}[\exp(-\theta \mathbf{X})]$. When no misunderstandings arise, we abbreviate this tedious expression by the shorter "the mgf of $\mathbf{X}$". For example, the mgf of a normal random variable X with mean μ and variance σ^2 is equal to

$$E[\exp(-\theta X)] = \int_{-\infty}^{\infty} \exp(-\theta x) \cdot \frac{1}{\sigma\sqrt{2\pi}} \exp\left[-\frac{1}{2}\left(\frac{(x-\mu)}{\sigma}\right)^2\right] dx$$

$$= \exp\left(-\mu\theta + \frac{1}{2}\sigma^2\theta^2\right) \tag{3.12}$$

Using similar limiting arguments as for the mean and variance of $X(t)$ that have led us to Eqs. (3.1)–(3.3), the moment-generating technique permits us to determine the mgf—and thus the distribution—of $X(t)$ from the mgf characterizing any single step.

Starting at $x_0 = 0$, the position of the walk at time Δt, after the first step, is with equal probability $+\Delta x$ or $-\Delta x$, and so the mgf of $X(\Delta t)$ equals

$$E[\exp(-\theta X(\Delta t))] = \frac{1}{2}\left[\exp(+\theta\Delta x) + \exp(-\theta\Delta x)\right] = \cosh(\theta\Delta x)$$

where $\cosh(z)$ is the hyperbolic cosine function.

Again, $X(t = n\Delta t)$ is the sum of $n = t/\Delta t$ independent steps. As described in Sect. 2.3.6 for pgfs, the mgf of a sum of n identical and independent random variables is the mgf of the individual summand, raised to the power n. Therefore, after $n = t/\Delta t$ steps have been carried out at time t

$$m_t(\theta) = E[\exp(-\theta X(t))] = \left[\cosh(\theta\sigma\sqrt{\Delta t})\right]^{\frac{t}{\Delta t}}$$

where we have inserted the limiting relation $\Delta x = \sigma\sqrt{\Delta t}$, as discussed in Eq. (3.3) above.

For the limit contemplated, we next replace our expression for $m_t(\theta)$ with the series representation $\cosh(z) \approx 1 + \frac{1}{2}z^2 + \ldots$, valid for small $z = \theta\sigma\sqrt{\Delta t}$. For small values of Δt, we thus obtain

$$m_t(\theta) \approx \left[1 + \frac{1}{2}\left(\theta\sigma\sqrt{\Delta t}\right)^2\right]^{\frac{t}{\Delta t}} = \left\{\left[1 + \frac{\frac{1}{2}(\theta\sigma)^2}{\frac{1}{\Delta t}}\right]^{\frac{1}{\Delta t}}\right\}^t$$

The expression in curly brackets has the general form $(1+\alpha/m)^m$, with $\alpha = \frac{1}{2}(\theta\sigma)^2$ and $m = 1/\Delta t$. For $\Delta t \to 0$, we have $m \to \infty$ and $(1 + \alpha/m)^m \to e^\alpha$. Taking the outer exponent t into account, we finally get for the limit indicated

$$m_t(\theta) = E[\exp(-\theta X(t))] = \exp\left[\frac{1}{2}\theta^2(\sigma^2 t)\right] \tag{3.13}$$

By comparison with Eq. (3.12), we recognize this to be the mgf of a normal distribution with mean $\mu = 0$ and variance $\sigma^2 t$. If the starting point is not 0 but more generally x_0, then the entire density is simply displaced by x_0, in agreement with Eq. (3.8).

3.4   Some Elementary Properties of the Continuous Limit

To gain more familiarity with the solution Eq. (3.8) of the forward and the backward diffusion equation, in this section, we look at a few elementary properties of the continuous limit of the simple symmetric random walk.

Let us assume that the process $X(t)$ starts at $x_0 = 0$ and first ask: which proportion of all realizations of $\{X(t), t \geq 0\}$—that is, of all sample paths described by $(t, X(t))$—will ever reach the level $a > 0$ at some time during the interval $[0, t]$? For example, we might simulate the diffusion process $\{X(t), t \geq 0\}$ a great number of times and count the relative frequency of those realizations in which the level a was reached at some time during the interval $[0, d]$. More formally, if we denote the *first-passage time* to the level a as the random variable $\mathbf{T}_a$, then that relative frequency will tend to $P(\mathbf{T}_a \leq d)$.

To address this question, we use an elementary symmetry argument, much like the one that we illustrated in Fig. 2.10 for correlated random walks and in Exercise 5 of Chap. 2. As illustrated by the path in Fig. 3.2 that starts at time $t = 0$ at $X(t) = 0$ and ends at time $t = 1000$ at $X(t) = 5$, any path which at time $t = 1000$ is above the level $a = 3$ (so that $X(t) > a$) must necessarily have crossed that level for the first time at some earlier time $0 < t' < t$. From the basic directional symmetry of the process, the transitions of this path are just as likely as those of the "mirror path" that before t' is identical to $X(t)$ and after t' takes the values $2a - X(t)$. The reason is that once a path has reached $X(t') = a$, it is equally likely that in the remaining interval $t - t'$, it will move to $a + x$ or to $a - x$. That is, for all paths that at time $t = 1000$ are above the level $a = 3$, we expect an equal number of paths that also had reached a but then again dropped below that level. For example, for the path in Fig. 3.2 that had reached $a = 3$ and ended at $X(t) = 5 = a + 2$ we expect another, equally likely path starting at $x = 0$ that had also reached $a = 3$ but ended at $X(t) = 1 = a - 2$. This heuristic argument gives

$$P(\mathbf{T}_a \leq t) = 2 \cdot P(X(t) > a) = 2 \cdot \left[1 - \Phi\left(\frac{a}{\sigma\sqrt{t}} \right) \right] = 2 \cdot \Phi\left(-\frac{a}{\sigma\sqrt{t}} \right)$$

because we already know from Eq. (3.8) that $X(t)$ has the normal distribution with mean 0 and variance $\sigma^2 t$.

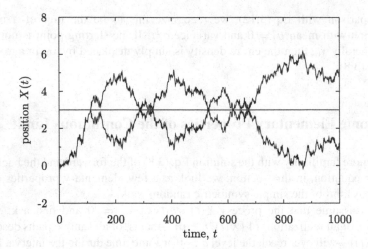

Fig. 3.2 The original path $X(t)$ starting at $x = 0$ passes the barrier at $a = 3$ (shown as a horizontal line) for the first time at $t = 112$ and ends at $x = 5$. The mirror path coincides with the original path till that moment and is from there on the reflection of the original path with respect to the line $a = 3$ (i.e., $2a - X(t)$); it thus ends at $x = 1$. From the basic directional symmetry of the process as characterized by Eq. (3.8), both paths are equally likely. Thus, for any path starting at $x = 0$ which at $t = 1000$ ends above the line at $x > a$, there will be another equally likely path starting at $x = 0$ which also reached the line $x = a$ but at $t = 1000$ ends at $2a - x$ below the line

Clearly, from the spatial homogeneity of the process, if the start is not at 0 but at $x_0 < a$, then all events are simply spatially displaced by this offset, and we get

$$P(\mathbf{T}_a \le t) = 2 \cdot \Phi\left(-\frac{a - x_0}{\sigma\sqrt{t}}\right) \qquad (3.14)$$

Differentiating Eq. (3.14) with respect to t, we find the corresponding density g of the first-passage time $\mathbf{T}_a$

$$g(t|a, x_0) = \frac{a - x_0}{\sigma\sqrt{2\pi t^3}} \cdot \exp\left[-\frac{(a - x_0)^2}{2\sigma^2 t}\right] \qquad (3.15)$$

Three typical examples of the density Eq. (3.15) appear in Fig. 3.3, which shows the influence of varying the barrier a or the variance σ^2. Note the thick tails to the right of $g(t|a, x_0)$ which leads to an infinite expectation of $\mathbf{T}_a$; we therefore look at alternative measures to characterize the central tendency of these first-passage times.

For example, we find the median first-passage time from Eq. (3.14) by setting $P(\mathbf{T}_a \le \tilde{t}) = \frac{1}{2}$; it is equal to $\tilde{t} = 2.20\left(\frac{a-x_0}{\sigma}\right)^2$. Similarly, the mode of the density Eq. (3.15) is obtained from the condition $g'(t_{mode}|a, x_0) = 0$; it is equal to $t_{mode} = \frac{1}{3}\left(\frac{a-x_0}{\sigma}\right)^2$. Thus, the mode is smaller than the median by a factor of more than 6, indicating the marked skew of the first-passage time distribution Eq. (3.15). Both

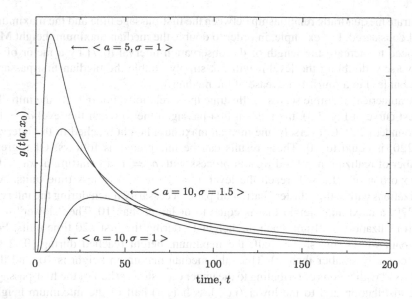

Fig. 3.3 Three first-passage time densities $g(t|a, x_0)$ as given by Eq. (3.15); all densities refer to a start point of $x_0 = 0$; abscissa, time, t; ordinate, density $g(t|a, x_0)$. Relative to the density of the slowest ($a = 10, \sigma = 1$) first-passage time, the leftmost density ($a = 5, \sigma = 1$) illustrates the speed-up due to a closer barrier and the middle density ($a = 10, \sigma = 1.5$) the speed-up due to a larger variance

measures of the central tendency describe the quadratic increase of $\mathbf{T}_a$ with the distance $a - x_0$ of the barrier a from the start at x_0. Also, as is clear from Eq. (3.14), multiplying all three parameters $< a, x_0, \sigma >$ by the same factor has no effect on the distribution of $\mathbf{T}_a$. This is intuitively obvious: we may project the entire process as shown in Fig. 3.2 onto a larger or smaller vertical spatial scale, but this would not affect the time at which the barrier is first reached.

A question closely related to the first-passage time $\mathbf{T}_a$ is: what is the distribution of the maximum height which a process governed by Eq. (3.8) starting at $x_0 = 0$ reaches during the interval $[0, t]$? Let us denote the maximum height in $[0, t]$ as the random variable $\mathbf{M}_t$. To address this question, we use an elementary one-to-one relation that exists between $\mathbf{M}_t$ and $\mathbf{T}_a$. That is, the maximum height $\mathbf{M}_t$ in $[0, t]$ is less than a if, and only if, the first passage to a takes place at a time later than t. Both statements express the same event: that the process $X(t)$ never reached the level a during the interval $[0, t]$. Using this equivalence, and our previous result Eq. (3.14)

$$P(\mathbf{M}_t < a) = P(\mathbf{T}_a > t) = 2 \cdot \Phi\left(\frac{a}{\sigma\sqrt{t}}\right) - 1 \qquad (3.16)$$

Based on Eq. (3.16), it is easy to calculate that the median maximum height $\mathbf{M}_t$ reached in $[0, t]$ is equal to $\tilde{a} = 0.6745\sigma\sqrt{t}$. Conversely, the median time until the level a is first reached is equal to $\tilde{t} = (a/0.6745\sigma)^2$. Both relations again illustrate the quadratic relationship between the first-passage time and the maximum level considered. For example, in order to double the median maximum height $\mathbf{M}_t$, we need to increase the length of the observation interval $[0, t]$ by a factor of 4. Conversely, doubling the level a will not simply double the median first-passage time but lead to a fourfold increase of the median $\mathbf{T}_a$.

A numerical example serves to illustrate these relations. For $\sigma = 1$ (the initially lowest curve in Fig. 3.3), the median first-passage time to reach the level $a = 10$ is (rounded) 220. Conversely, the median maximum height reached in the interval $[0, 220]$ is equal to 10. These results can be interpreted as follows. Of a great number of realizations of a diffusion process with $\sigma = 1$, all starting at $x_0 = 0$, a proportion of 50% will reach the level $a = 10$ in 220 or less time units. All realizations within this "faster" half of all paths necessarily reach during the interval $[0, 220]$ a maximum height that is equal to or larger than 10. The "slower" half of all realizations will not reach the height 10 during the first 220 time units. For any path within this slower half, the maximum height reached during $[0, 220]$ is necessarily smaller than 10. Thus, the median maximum height is 10, and the subsets of realizations contributing to the upper (i.e., slower) half of the first-passage time distribution and to the lower (i.e., less height) half of the maximum height distribution are exactly the same.

In 1918, the physicist Philipp Frank proposed an interesting alternative notion of the speed of propagation of diffusion processes as they arise as limits of simple symmetric random walks. Frank imagined a large number m of independent particles, all starting at $t = 0$ from $x_0 = 0$. According to Eq. (3.8), at time t, the probability is then $1 - \Phi\left(\frac{a}{\sigma\sqrt{t}}\right)$ that an individual particle happens to be above the level a. Therefore, if a_m is chosen such that $1 - \Phi\left(\frac{a_m}{\sigma\sqrt{t}}\right) = \frac{1}{m}$, then we have implicitly defined a level a_m that at time t will on average be exceeded by exactly one—called the "head of the swarm" by Frank—of all m particles. For example, for $t = 1$ and $\sigma = 1$, this critical level is $a_m = 3.09$ for $m = 1000$ particles, which indicates that at time $t = 1$ on average, only 1 of 1000 particles will be found above the level $a_m = 3.09$.

At the same time, we may register the maximum height reached by each of these 1000 particles in $[0, 1]$ individually and then look at the largest of these maximum heights—which represents the highest position that had been reached by any particle at any time in $[0, 1]$. As we concluded from Eq. (3.16), the median of the maximum heights $\mathbf{M}_t$ reached in $[0, 1]$ by the particles is then equal to just 0.6745. However, the median of the largest maximum height of $m = 1000$ particles all moving independently is about 3.393. Thus, although at $t = 1$ we expect on average only one particle above the level $a = 3.09$, the median largest excursion that had been reached by any particle at any time during the interval $[0, 1]$ is quite a bit larger. Section 7.5 describes a related application of these concepts to the evolution of scores during sport matches, which also contrasts the final level of a random process with its maximum interim level.

3.5 Exercises

1. Using Eq. (3.8) with $x_0 = 0$ for the density f, show that the probability flux through x at time t may be written as

$$J(x, t) = f(x, t) \frac{x}{2t}$$

Comment upon the form of $J(x, t)$ when x is negative, zero, and positive and for small vs. large t. Show that at time t the (absolute) flux is maximal at $x = \pm\sigma\sqrt{t}$. Why is this in accordance with Fick's law?

2. Explain why even though three parameters $(a, x_0,$ and $\sigma)$ appear in Eq. (3.15) the density g essentially depends only on a single parameter and may in any case be normalized as

$$g^*(t|\alpha) = \frac{\alpha}{\sqrt{2\pi t^3}} \cdot \exp\left(-\frac{\alpha^2}{2t}\right)$$

where $\alpha = (a - x_0)/\sigma > 0$.

3. When starting at $x_0 = 0$, the mgf of the first-passage time $\mathbf{T}_a$ to the level a may be shown to be

$$m(\theta) = \mathsf{E}[\exp(-\theta \mathbf{T}_a)] = \exp\left(-\frac{a}{\sigma}\sqrt{2\theta}\right)$$

Based on the form of m, argue that the sum of n independent random variables $\mathbf{T}_a$ is distributed as is the random variable $n^2 \cdot \mathbf{T}_a$. Observe that the sum of n independent random variables $\mathbf{T}_a$ may be interpreted as $\mathbf{T}_{na}$, the first-passage time through the level na. Argue from Eq. (3.14) for $x_0 = 0$ that the distribution of $\mathbf{T}_{na}$ is the same as the distribution of $n^2 \cdot \mathbf{T}_a$. For example, doubling the threshold level a will increase the first-passage time by a factor of 4.

4. Give a probabilistic interpretation of the fact that for all a and $\sigma > 0$, it is true that for $\theta = 0$, the mgf equals $m(0) = 1$. Relate this property to our previous finding Eq. (2.9) for simple random walks with $p = \frac{1}{2}$.

5. For $x_0 = 0$, show that if the random variable $\mathbf{T}_a$ has the density Eq. (3.15), then its reciprocal $1/\mathbf{T}_a$ is distributed as $(\sigma/a)^2 \chi_1^2$ where χ_1^2 is a chi-square random variable with $df = 1$. For example, its expectation is $\mathsf{E}[1/\mathbf{T}_a] = \mathsf{E}[(\sigma/a)^2 \chi_1^2] = (\sigma/a)^2$; explain why this expectation increases with σ and decreases with a.

6. In analogy to the usual notion of speed as distance divided by the time needed to cover that distance, a simple measure of the "speed" of the process $\{X(t)\}$ might be the quantity $a/\mathbf{T}_a$. In view of Exercise 5, would this be a sensible measure?

7. Assume that a correlated random walk (Sect. 2.4) starts with equal probability in an upward or downward directional state $(g = \frac{1}{2}$, in the terminology of Sect. 2.4.4), in which case the mean of the position after n steps is generally 0, and so the variance is given by Eq. (2.41). Consider a limit process for small

$\Delta t \rightarrow 0$ such that the local speed $\Delta x / \Delta t = v$ remains constant. Given the basic symmetry of the transition matrix Eq. (2.32) of a correlated random walk, for any fixed $p < 1$, the process would degenerate to a deterministic horizontal movement $x(t) = 0$ as $\Delta t \rightarrow 0$. However, when $p \rightarrow 1$, rigidly persistent transitions may counterbalance the inherently equalizing effect of an increasing number of steps per fixed time interval $[0, t]$; this balance may be obtained by coupling the persistence parameter p to Δt such that $p = 1 - \frac{\beta}{2}\Delta t$. Show that under this scenario, the variance Eq. (2.41) of the process after $t = n\Delta t$ time units tends to

$$\text{Var}[X(t)] = \frac{2v^2}{\beta^2} \left(\beta t + \exp(-\beta t) - 1 \right)$$

Consider and explain the two quite different regimes of $\text{Var}[X(t)]$ for small and large t.

8. Show how Eq. (3.5) can be obtained from Eq. (3.4) by noting that f'' is the derivative of f'.

Chapter 4
Diffusion with Drift: The Wiener Process

In Chap. 3, we studied a limiting process in which the duration Δt and the size Δx of the steps of a simple symmetric random walk both decrease toward zero. Under specific conditions, such as Eq. (3.3), this process tends in the limit to a continuous diffusion process that is governed by the time-dependent state density as given by Eq. (3.8). Just as the simple symmetric random walk has no systematic tendency to move upward or downward (cf., Eq. (2.1)), so Eq. (3.8) indicates that in the limiting diffusion process, we have $\mathsf{E}[X(t)] = x_0$ for all t. Clearly, this feature is too rigid in many contexts in which we are specifically interested in the accumulation of systematic changes in the state space across time.

To overcome this conceptual limitation, in this section, we study the corresponding limiting diffusion process for a simple, but not necessarily symmetric, random walk. A diffusion process with constant drift and variance is called a Wiener process.[1] It is related to the simple diffusion process considered in Sect. 3 in the same way as is a discrete random walk with asymmetrical step probability $p \neq \frac{1}{2}$ to a symmetrical random walk, $p = \frac{1}{2}$.

In many applied fields, the Wiener process is the standard model of diffusive processes showing a systematic drift component. In diffusion-based modeling in the behavioral and life sciences, it plays a central role, in much the same way as the normal-error general linear model with its techniques of regression, correlation, and analysis of variance plays a central role in many fields applying standard statistical analyses. One important reason for this prominence is that, on the one hand, the Wiener process offers sufficient structure to capture critical conceptual aspects and thus to serve as a plausible initial model in a diverse range of applications. At the same time, it is still manageable enough so that tractable explicit analytic solutions can be found, which is not the case for many of the more complex diffusion models.

---

[1] After the mathematician Norbert Wiener (1894–1964).

© Springer Nature Switzerland AG 2022
W. Schwarz, *Random Walk and Diffusion Models*,
https://doi.org/10.1007/978-3-031-12100-5_4

The present chapter describes and explains basic features and applicable results related to this standard model of diffusion processes.

4.1 Unrestricted Evolution

4.1.1 Limit Conditions for Discrete Random Walks with Drift

In Chap. 3, we have seen that simple diffusion processes may be understood as a limit of discrete random walks, carrying out steps of sizes tending to zero but at a very high speed. In particular, we have seen that discrete random walks with no drift may admit a meaningful limit for steps of decreasing size and decreasing duration—given that the limiting process considered satisfies certain conditions. More specifically, according to Eq. (3.3), the size Δx and duration Δt of the steps must tend to zero in a way such that $\lim_{\substack{\Delta t \to 0 \\ \Delta x \to 0}} \frac{(\Delta x)^2}{\Delta t} \to \sigma^2 > 0$. In effect, this means that the step size must in the limit be such that $\Delta x = \sigma \sqrt{\Delta t}$.

Which modifications of these conditions are required when $p \neq \frac{1}{2}$ so that according to Eq. (2.1) the random walk has nonzero drift? Each single step will then with probability p lead $+\Delta x$ units upward and with probability $1 - p$ lead $-\Delta x$ units downward. The expected displacement after a single step, at time Δt, is therefore

$$E[X(\Delta t)] = (+\Delta x) \cdot p + (-\Delta x) \cdot (1 - p) = (2p - 1)\,\Delta x \qquad (4.1)$$

Similarly, the variance of the displacement after a single step is

$$\text{Var}[X(\Delta t)] = E[X^2(\Delta t)] - E^2[X(\Delta t)] = 4p(1 - p)\,(\Delta x)^2 \qquad (4.2)$$

Therefore, at time t, after $n = t/\Delta t$ independent steps have been completed, the mean and variance of the position of the walk are given by

$$E[X(t = n\Delta t)] = n\,(2p - 1)\,\Delta x = t\,(2p - 1)\,\frac{\Delta x}{\Delta t} \qquad (4.3)$$

and

$$\text{Var}[X(t = n\Delta t)] = n\,4p(1 - p)\,(\Delta x)^2 = t\,4p(1 - p)\,\frac{(\Delta x)^2}{\Delta t} \qquad (4.4)$$

As in the drift-free case of $p = \frac{1}{2}$, Eq. (4.4) requires that Δt and Δx jointly tend to zero such that in the limit $\frac{(\Delta x)^2}{\Delta t} \to \sigma^2$. On inserting this relation into Eq. (4.3), we see that $E[X(t)]$ is proportional to $(2p - 1)\frac{1}{\Delta x}$.

In the presence of nonzero drift, Eq. (4.3) implies an additional requirement concerning the step probabilities p. Namely, as the size and the duration of the steps decrease, p must remain close to $\frac{1}{2}$ because only then will the expression $(2p - 1)\frac{1}{\Delta x}$ to which $\mathsf{E}[X(t)]$ is proportional remain bounded. This feature reflects that when the number of steps per time unit gets very large, any rigidly set value of $p \neq \frac{1}{2}$ such as, say, $p = 0.52$ would vault the process beyond any given limit. Equation (4.3) suggests that $\mathsf{E}[X(t)]$ will tend to a meaningful continuous limit if the step probabilities p vary with decreasing Δt and Δx such that $2p - 1 \propto \Delta x$ as Δt and Δx tend to zero. Therefore, remembering that $\Delta x = \sigma\sqrt{\Delta t}$, if we set $p = \frac{1}{2}(1 + \frac{\mu}{\sigma}\sqrt{\Delta t})$, where μ is a constant whose interpretation we consider below, then we will have $2p - 1 = \frac{\mu}{\sigma}\sqrt{\Delta t}$ and $4p(1 - p) = 1 - \frac{\mu^2}{\sigma^2}\Delta t$. Inserting these relations into Equations 4.3 and 4.4, we get

$$\mathsf{E}[X(t)] = t\,(2p - 1)\frac{\Delta x}{\Delta t} = t\,\frac{\mu}{\sigma}\sqrt{\frac{(\Delta x)^2}{\Delta t}} \tag{4.5}$$

and also

$$\mathsf{Var}[X(t)] = t\left(1 - \frac{\mu^2}{\sigma^2}\Delta t\right)\frac{(\Delta x)^2}{\Delta t} \tag{4.6}$$

Looking now at the limit $\lim_{\substack{\Delta t \to 0 \\ \Delta x \to 0}} \frac{(\Delta x)^2}{\Delta t} \to \sigma^2$, we then obtain

$$\mathsf{E}[X(t)] = \mu t \tag{4.7}$$

Thus, the constant μ is seen to be the mean displacement of $X(t)$ per time unit. Also, for the limit indicated, we get from Eq. (4.6) as in the case of $p = \frac{1}{2}$

$$\mathsf{Var}[X(t)] = \sigma^2 t \tag{4.8}$$

In summary, if in a simple random walk the durations Δt and the (absolute) sizes Δx of the steps tend to zero, then the walk may tend to a continuous diffusion process $X(t)$ in which the mean and variance are proportional to t, that is, $\mathsf{E}[X(t)] = \mu t$ and $\mathsf{Var}[X(t)] = \sigma^2 t$. However, this limit requires specific assumptions about the relative rates with which Δt and Δx tend to zero. One condition to obtain this convergence is that in the limit of $\Delta t \to 0$ and $\Delta x \to 0$, we have

$$\lim_{\substack{\Delta t \to 0 \\ \Delta x \to 0}} \frac{(\Delta x)^2}{\Delta t} \to \sigma^2 \quad \text{and} \quad p(\Delta x, \Delta t) = \frac{1}{2}(1 + \frac{\mu}{\sigma}\sqrt{\Delta t}) \tag{4.9}$$

4.1.2   The Forward Equation in the Presence of Drift

In Sect. 3.2.2, we have seen that the basic forward Equation (3.7), and its appropriate solution Eq. (3.8), naturally flows from the two Fick assumptions regarding the nature of physical diffusion processes, discussed in Sect. 1.2.2. These results correspond to one interpretation of the continuous limit of balls undergoing a simple symmetric random walk as they pass through Galton's board.

Fick's assumptions refer to the case of "pure diffusion", when no external forces act upon the movement of the particles (Fig. 1.5). What changes in this approach if external forces acting on the process are present, in addition to pure diffusion? In this section, we consider the case of a spatially and temporally *uniform* force, such as gravitation is in physical applications. That is, we consider a force which acts in the same manner at any position x and at any time t. As before, we will use the metaphorical Fick terminology of a diffusing substance, thought of as a great number of diffusing particles.

In the presence of a uniform force μ, acting into the positive x—direction—that is, from left-to-right for positive μ—the generalized Fick law states that the amount of substance passing in a small time interval $[t, t + \Delta t]$ through a cross-section at x is additively composed of the "pure" diffusion stream, plus the amount of substance passing due to the (constant) external force, μ. The assumptions concerning the pure diffusion stream are exactly the same as before (cf., Sect. 1.2.2). The component of change due to the external force corresponds to ordinary deterministic particle movement.

How does this translate to the situation of a random walk with drift? Consider again the events on a Galton board (Fig. 1.3) at a position x in a small time interval $[t, t + \Delta t]$. The uniform force just mentioned is represented by the constant drift $2p - 1$ (cf., Sect. 2.2 or Eq. (4.1)) in the simple random walk for which Galton's board represents a physical analogy. In terms of Fig. 1.3, we assume that upon reaching the tip of a wedge, the balls fall with a probability of p to the right and with probability $1 - p$ to the left.

Corresponding to our approach and notation in Sect. 3.2.2, let the distribution function $F(x, t)$ represent the fraction of balls to the left of x at time t (where t corresponds to the vertical axis, the height of the row in Fig. 1.3), and let $f(x, t)$ be the corresponding local density, $f(x, t) = \frac{\partial F}{\partial x}$. Therefore, at time (row) t, a fraction of about $F(x, t) - F(x - \Delta x, t) \approx f(x - \Delta x/2, t)\Delta x$ of all balls emanating at $t = 0$ from the funnel will be found in the small interval $[x - \Delta x, x]$. During the time interval $[t, t + \Delta t]$, a fraction of p of these balls will move one spatial step Δx to the right and therefore *exit* the region below x, representing the *outflow* from the region below x.

Similarly, at time t, a fraction of $F(x + \Delta x, t) - F(x, t) \approx f(x + \Delta x/2, t)\Delta x$ balls will be found in the adjacent small interval $[x, x + \Delta x]$. Of these, a fraction of $1 - p$ will move during the time interval $[t, t + \Delta t]$ considered to the left, that is, *enter* the region below x from the right. This component represents the *inflow* into the region below x. In a small interval $[t, t + \Delta t]$, more distant balls will not cross the level x.

The net change of the fraction of balls below x in this time interval will thus be

$$\text{inflow} - \text{outflow} = (1 - p) f(x + \Delta x/2, t)\Delta x - p f(x - \Delta x/2, t)\Delta x$$

We next rewrite the right-hand side in the form

$$p\left[f(x + \Delta x/2, t) - f(x - \Delta x/2, t)\right]\Delta x \quad - \quad (2p - 1) f(x + \Delta x/2, t)\Delta x$$

We have seen that for a meaningful limit to exist for small Δx and Δt, we must have $\Delta x = \sigma\sqrt{\Delta t}$ and that $p \to \frac{1}{2}$ such that $(2p - 1) \to \frac{\mu}{\sigma}\sqrt{\Delta t} = \frac{\mu}{\sigma^2}\Delta x$. We also know from Sect. 3.2.1 that for small Δx such as we are considering, we have $f(x + \Delta x/2, t) - f(x - \Delta x/2, t) \approx \frac{\partial}{\partial x} f(x, t) \Delta x$. Inserting these relations gives for the inflow minus outflow relation

$$\text{inflow} - \text{outflow} \approx p\frac{\partial}{\partial x} f(x, t)(\Delta x)^2 - \frac{\mu}{\sigma^2} f(x + \Delta x/2, t)(\Delta x)^2$$

Given the local nature of the movements involved (i.e., balls further away from x cannot contribute to the local change at x during $[t, t + \Delta t]$), this change also corresponds to the change in the proportion of balls to the left of x in $[t, t + \Delta t]$. Thus, again appealing to the approximation of differences by derivatives explained in Sect. 3.2.1, we get

$$F(x, t + \Delta t) - F(x, t) \approx \Delta t \frac{\partial}{\partial t} F(x, t) \quad =$$

$$p\frac{\partial}{\partial x} f(x, t)(\Delta x)^2 - \frac{\mu}{\sigma^2} f(x + \Delta x/2, t)(\Delta x)^2 \tag{4.10}$$

$F(x, t)$ is the distribution function giving the proportion of balls to the left of x at time t, so its derivative with respect to x is the corresponding density $f(x, t)$ at time t. Differentiating both sides of Eq. (4.10) with respect to x and dividing by Δt give

$$\frac{\partial}{\partial t} f(x, t) = p\frac{\partial^2}{\partial x^2} f(x, t)\frac{(\Delta x)^2}{\Delta t} - \frac{\mu}{\sigma^2}\frac{\partial}{\partial x} f(x + \Delta x/2, t)\frac{(\Delta x)^2}{\Delta t} \tag{4.11}$$

Now going as before to the limit $\Delta t \to 0$ and $\Delta x \to 0$ so that

$$\lim_{\substack{\Delta t \to 0 \\ \Delta x \to 0}} \frac{(\Delta x)^2}{\Delta t} \to \sigma^2 \quad \text{and} \quad \lim_{\substack{\Delta t \to 0 \\ \Delta x \to 0}} p = p(\Delta x, \Delta t) = \frac{1}{2}$$

we get

$$\frac{\partial}{\partial t} f(x, t) = \frac{1}{2}\sigma^2 \frac{\partial^2}{\partial x^2} f(x, t) - \mu \frac{\partial}{\partial x} f(x, t) \tag{4.12}$$

the forward diffusion equation for a constant force, μ. As expected, in the absence
of any external force ($\mu = 0$), Eq. (4.12) reduces to Eq. (3.7).

The distribution function $F(x, t)$ is the probability for a single ball to be to the
left of x at time t. Therefore, if we divide both sides of Eq. (4.10) by Δt, we get the
total change $F(x, t + \Delta t) - F(x, t)$ of probability content to the left of x per time
unit during the interval $[t, t + \Delta t]$—the net flux of probability across the coordinate
x. Using the same assumptions and operations as above, for small steps and short
durations, the limit indicated is seen after dividing Eq. (4.10) by Δt to be equal to

$$\frac{\partial}{\partial t} F(x, t) = \frac{1}{2} \sigma^2 \frac{\partial}{\partial x} f(x, t) - \mu f(x, t)$$

We already noticed in the derivation of the local flux at t for the drift-free case,
Eq. (3.11), that in the way indicated, the direction of the flux would be taken from
right to left. This is because the expression for it in Eq. (4.10) is positive when
$F(x, t + \Delta t) > F(x, t)$, that is, when more balls are below x at time $t + \Delta t$ than
there were at time t. If, more conventionally, the flux is taken in the positive, left-
to-right direction, a negative sign must precede this expression. This produces the
standard form for the left-to-right flux $J(x, t)$ of probability at t across x

$$J(x, t) = -\frac{1}{2} \sigma^2 \frac{\partial}{\partial x} f(x, t) + \mu f(x, t) \qquad (4.13)$$

We have seen (Eq. (3.11)) that in a pure diffusion process, at time t, the amount
$J(x, t)$ of substance passing through a cross-section at x is proportional to the
gradient of concentration at x, that is, to $\frac{\partial}{\partial x} f(x, t)$, which is just another form
to express the second assumption of Fick, described in Sect. 1.2.2. In the presence
of an additional external force acting on the process, a further component is added
to the flux. According to Eq. (4.13), this additional component is proportional to the
current local concentration f of substance (balls) at x and to the magnitude and
direction of the external force, μ. For example, if μ is positive, then there will, in
addition to the purely diffusive movement, arise a further flux component across x in
the left-to-right direction that is larger the larger the μ and the larger the current local
concentration $f(x, t)$ is. We will return to the notion of the flux of probability across
x when we discuss boundary conditions for absorbing (Sect. 4.2.1) and reflecting
(Sect. 4.3) barriers delimiting the Wiener diffusion process.

4.1.3 The Backward Equation for the Wiener Process

In Sect. 2.2.2, we have seen that by conditioning on the outcome of the first step,
we can derive an equation—the backward Eq. (2.4)—that describes the evolution
of a discrete simple random walk. Taking the appropriate limits for small steps
of short duration (cf., Eq. (3.3)), the backward Eq. (3.9) for the transition density

$f(x_0, x, t)$ of a drift-free diffusion process represents the continuous counterpart to the backward Eq. (2.4) for a symmetric simple random walk. We now aim at a comparable backward equation for $f(x_0, x, t)$ for the Wiener process, that is, in the presence of a constant drift term.

Consider, then, a random walk starting at $t = 0$ at position $x_0 = k\Delta x$. Denote as $f[k\Delta x, x, (n + 1)\Delta t]$ the probability for the walk to be at position x after $(n + 1)$ steps, when each step has duration Δt and (absolute) size Δx. Clearly, f depends on the final level x, but to simplify our notation and to focus on quantities that actually vary, we suppress this constant final level for the moment, writing for short $f(x_0, x, t) = f(x_0, t)$. As before, our aim is to study f in the limit of Eq. (3.3)

$$\lim_{\substack{\Delta t \to 0 \\ \Delta x \to 0}} \frac{(\Delta x)^2}{\Delta t} \to \sigma^2 \quad \text{and} \quad p(\Delta x, \Delta t) = \frac{1}{2}\left(1 + \frac{\mu}{\sigma}\sqrt{\Delta t}\right)$$

The first step takes the walk either (with probability p) to position $(k + 1)\Delta x$ or (probability $1 - p$) to position $(k - 1)\Delta x$. The basic recursion, then, is

$$f[k\Delta x, (n + 1)\Delta t] = p \cdot f[(k + 1)\Delta x, n\Delta t] + (1 - p) \cdot f[(k - 1)\Delta x, n\Delta t]$$

$$= \frac{1}{2}\left\{ f[(k + 1)\Delta x, n\Delta t] + f[(k - 1)\Delta x, n\Delta t]\right\} +$$

$$\frac{1}{2}\frac{\mu}{\sigma}\sqrt{\Delta t}\left\{ f[(k + 1)\Delta x, n\Delta t] - f[(k - 1)\Delta x, n\Delta t]\right\} \tag{4.14}$$

where the last two lines result upon inserting the relation $p = \frac{1}{2}\left(1 + \frac{\mu}{\sigma}\sqrt{\Delta t}\right)$, then separating the terms corresponding to $\frac{1}{2}$ and to $\frac{\mu}{2\sigma}\sqrt{\Delta t}$. We next subtract $f(k\Delta x, n\Delta t)$ on both sides of Eq. (4.14) and then divide through by $\Delta t = (\Delta x/\sigma)^2$. This gives

$$\frac{1}{\Delta t}[f(k\Delta x, (n + 1)\Delta t) - f(k\Delta x, n\Delta t)] =$$

$$\frac{1}{2}\sigma^2\frac{1}{(\Delta x)^2}\left\{ f[(k + 1)\Delta x, n\Delta t] - 2f[k\Delta x, n\Delta t] + f[(k - 1)\Delta x, n\Delta t]\right\} +$$

$$\mu\frac{1}{2\Delta x}\left\{ f[(k + 1)\Delta x, n\Delta t] - f[(k - 1)\Delta x, n\Delta t]\right\} \tag{4.15}$$

We now consider the indicated limits, much as we did in the case of no drift in Sect. 3.2.1. As before, the left-hand side of Eq. (4.15) clearly tends to $\frac{\partial f}{\partial t}$. The first summand on the right-hand side of Eq. (4.15) contains a second-order difference quotient and so according to Eq. (3.5) tends to $\frac{1}{2}\sigma^2\frac{\partial^2 f}{\partial x_0^2}$. Similarly, the second summand on the right-hand side of Eq. (4.15) contains a first-order difference quotient, with arguments separated by $2\Delta x$; following Eq. (3.4), it tends in the limit to $\mu\frac{\partial f}{\partial x_0}$. Together, then, writing more explicitly $f(x_0, x, t) = f(x_0, t)$, we get the backward equation for the Wiener process with drift

$$\frac{\partial f(x_0, x, t)}{\partial t} = \frac{1}{2}\sigma^2 \cdot \frac{\partial^2 f(x_0, x, t)}{\partial x_0^2} + \mu \cdot \frac{\partial f(x_0, x, t)}{\partial x_0} \qquad (4.16)$$

It is instructive to compare Eqs. (4.12) and 4.16 for the same transition density $f(x_0, x, t)$. Both equations relate the first-order temporal derivative to a spatial variable: Eq. (4.12) refers to a fixed starting point x_0 and a variable level x; in contrast, Eq. (4.16) refers to a variable starting point x_0 and a fixed level x. Both versions are the more natural formulation in different contexts, but the backward Equation (4.16) is especially useful when we turn to first-passage time problems (cf., Sect. 4.2.2 and Chap. 6).

4.1.4 Explicit Form of the Transition Density

The solution of Eqs. (4.12) and (4.16) when a unit substance (i.e., with probability 1) is initially concentrated at x_0 is given by

$$f(x_0, x, t) = \frac{1}{\sigma\sqrt{2\pi t}} \cdot \exp\left[-\frac{(x - x_0 - \mu t)^2}{2\sigma^2 t}\right] \qquad (4.17)$$

The result Eq. (4.17) is basic and instructive; in many applications, $f(x_0, x, t)$ essentially forms the basis to address more specific aspects of the Wiener diffusion process, much in the way illustrated in Sect. 3.4. Note again the different conceptual meaning of the arguments x and t: the variable x refers to the values of the random variable $X(t)$, denoting the state (position) of the process at time t, whereas t is a fixed time index in Eq. (4.17). That is, for any t, the function f represents a probability density in the variable x that integrates to 1 across all (real) values of x. Specifically, Eq. (4.17) shows that for any t, the position $X(t)$ follows a normal distribution, with mean $E[X(t)] = x_0 + \mu t$ and variance $Var[X(t)] = \sigma^2 t$. The function f is called the *transition density* of a Wiener diffusion process to be at position x at time t when at time $t = 0$, it was at position x_0. It follows from the temporal homogeneity of the Wiener process that for any time interval of length t, the displacement $X(v+t) - X(v)$ is normally distributed with mean μt and variance $\sigma^2 t$, independent of $v \geq 0$.

In view of Sect. 4.1.1, this result may be understood as another example of the central limit theorem. Underlying the limiting process involving small steps of short duration is the idea that many independent steps of small size combine additively to determine the position of the process at any time. These are exactly the conditions under which the central limit theorem applies.

The result Eq. (4.17) also makes clear that the Wiener process can be interpreted as the superposition of deterministic linear movement with displacement μ per time unit and of a purely diffusive component as characterized by the variance parameter σ^2. If $\mu \to 0$, then we get the case of pure diffusion studied in Chap. 3. On the other hand, for $\sigma \to 0$, the process approaches standard deterministic movement of the type $y(t) = x_0 + \mu t$, where the drift μ plays the role of the constant velocity.

4.2 One Absorbing Barrier

In many applications of diffusion models, interest focuses on situations in which the state space of the process is delimited by one or two barriers. The practically most important example thereof are *absorbing* barriers. Conceptually, they correspond to the type of barriers that we have studied in Sect. 2.3 in some detail for discrete random walks and again in Sect. 2.4.3 for correlated random walks. If and when the process arrives at an absorbing barrier, it will not leave this state again. Important questions refer to the probability that a diffusion process ever reaches a given barrier and to the time it takes to reach it, given it ever arrives at that barrier. Another type of limitation of the state space that we will look at are barriers at which the process is *reflected*, much like a ball thrown against a wall.

The problem of the first-passage time density for the Wiener process in the presence of a single absorbing barrier is basic, and it illustrates very clearly several conceptual approaches that we can take to solve it. For two barriers, and for more complex diffusion processes, the central ideas remain essentially the same, but the technical problems then tend to dominate and to cloud the key points. Therefore, we will present three standard approaches to solve the first-passage time problem for the Wiener process, based on i.) the forward Equation (4.12), ii.) the backward Equation (4.16), and iii.) a limit process of the simple random walk.

4.2.1 The Forward Equation for First-Passage Times

Let $f(x_0, x, t | a)$ be the transition density of a Wiener process $\{X(t), t \geq 0\}$ with positive drift $\mu > 0$ starting at x_0 in the presence of an absorbing barrier at $a > x_0$, that is, f is the density for $X(t)$ to be at position $x < a$ at time $t > 0$.

Note that f is not simply the corresponding transition density for the case of unrestricted diffusion, that is, Eq. (4.17). For example, f obviously depends on the choice of a, whereas Eq. (4.17) does not. However, as regards the states below the level a, the "local" dynamics is still the same as in the absence of the barrier. For example, contemplating small changes of x and t, the same local limiting operations that we used in Sect. 4.1.2 would remain valid. Thus, even in the presence of a

barrier at $x = a$, for $x < a$, the transition density f still satisfies the forward
Equation (4.12)

$$\frac{\partial f(x_0, x, t|a)}{\partial t} = \frac{1}{2}\sigma^2 \cdot \frac{\partial^2 f(x_0, x, t|a)}{\partial x^2} - \mu \cdot \frac{\partial f(x_0, x, t|a)}{\partial x} \qquad (4.18)$$

where as before, f must be entirely concentrated at x_0 as $t \to 0$. Note that Eq. (4.18)
relates changes in t to those in x, whereas the starting point $x_0 < a$ remains constant.
Therefore, we focus for now on the case $x_0 = 0$ (as x_0 is a constant in the forward
equation), writing more compactly $f(x, t|a)$ to simplify our notation.

The notion of an absorbing barrier at $x = a$ means that the density $f(x, t|a)$ at
$x = a$ must vanish: in terms of Galton's board, as was shown in Fig. 1.4, all balls
arriving at $x = a$ are eliminated, and in terms of Fick's laws, all substance arriving
there sticks firmly to the wall at a. Technically, the density f at $x = a$ must be equal
to zero at all times t which is a form of a *boundary condition* imposed in addition
to the basic forward diffusion Equation (4.18). Thus, we next need to find a solution
to Eq. (4.18) which also satisfies the boundary condition

$$f(a, t|a) = 0 \qquad \text{for } t > 0 \qquad (4.19)$$

Note that the transition density f as given in Eq. (4.17) does satisfy the basic
forward equation; obviously, though, it does *not* satisfy the boundary condition
Eq. (4.19) imposed at $x = a$. However, we observe that if f satisfies the forward
diffusion Equation (4.18), then so does the function $f^*(x, t) = c \cdot f(x - k, t)$ and
thus also their sum, $f + f^*$. Therefore, we are free to determine a multiplicative
factor c and a shift constant k in a way such that the additional boundary condition
Eq. (4.19) at $x = a$ is satisfied. As we explain below, this approach produces the
specific solution of Eq. (4.18) that also satisfies boundary condition Eq. (4.19)

$$f(x, t|a) = \frac{1}{\sigma\sqrt{2\pi t}} \left\{ \exp\left[-\frac{(x - \mu t)^2}{2\sigma^2 t} \right] \right.$$

$$\left. - \exp\left(\frac{2\mu a}{\sigma^2} \right) \exp\left[-\frac{(x - 2a - \mu t)^2}{2\sigma^2 t} \right] \right\} \qquad (4.20)$$

In particular, inserting at $x = a$, we see that $f(a, t|a) = 0$ for all $t > 0$. For $\mu = 0$,
Eq. (4.20) represents the direct continuous counterpart to the discrete probabilities
$p_a(i, n)$ obtained for simple random walks in Exercise 6 of Chap. 2.

How does one arrive at this solution? The basis is the elementary algebraic
identity

$$(a - \mu t)^2 = -4a\mu t + (a + \mu t)^2$$

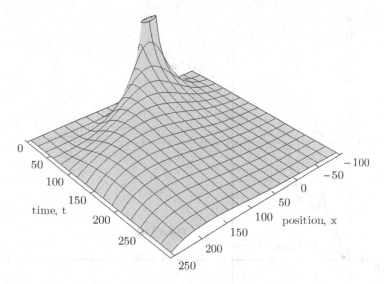

Fig. 4.1 The evolution of the transition density $f(x, t|a)$ of a Wiener process in the presence of an absorbing barrier at $a = 250$, for $\mu = 1, \sigma = 8$ during the time interval $[0, 250]$. Left axis, time t; right axis, spatial position x of the process; vertical axis, density $f(x, t|a)$; the absorbing barrier a is placed at the spatial coordinate $x = 250$

Dividing both sides by $-2\sigma^2 t$, we get, using $(a + \mu t)^2 = (-a - \mu t)^2$,

$$-\frac{(a - \mu t)^2}{2\sigma^2 t} = \frac{2a\mu}{\sigma^2} - \frac{(-a - \mu t)^2}{2\sigma^2 t}$$

Exponentiating, then dividing both sides by $\sigma \sqrt{2\pi t}$, we have

$$\frac{1}{\sigma \sqrt{2\pi t}} \exp\left[-\frac{(a - \mu t)^2}{2\sigma^2 t}\right] = \frac{1}{\sigma \sqrt{2\pi t}} \exp\left(\frac{2\mu a}{\sigma^2}\right) \exp\left[-\frac{(-a - \mu t)^2}{2\sigma^2 t}\right]$$

The two sides of this equation correspond precisely to the two summands of the solution Eq. (4.20), evaluated at $x = a$, showing that $f(a, t) = 0$ for all t.

Figure 4.1 shows the transition density $f(x, t|a)$ for $\mu = 1, \sigma = 8$, and $a = 250$. For small t, the entire probability mass is concentrated near $x_0 = 0$. The subsequent spreading shows the systematic drift toward positive states. Probability mass flows off across the barrier at $a = 250$, and so less probability mass is covered by f as t increases. For example, as hinted at in the foreground of Fig. 4.1, for $t = 250$, the density f covers only a mass of about 0.405 any more. As shown along the t−axis to the left, observe that $f = 0$ at $x = a = 250$ at all times t, as required by Eq. (4.19).

It is important to understand the conceptual nature of the transition density $f(x, t|a)$, as illustrated in Fig. 4.2. It represents the density of the process to be

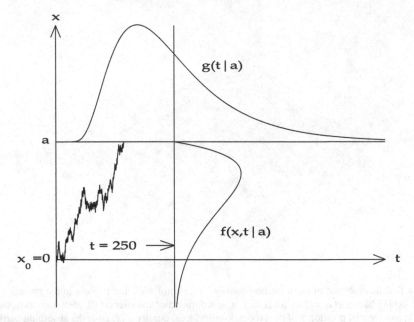

Fig. 4.2   The relation of the transition density $f(x, t|a)$ to the first-passage time density $g(t|a)$. A sample path starting at $x_0 = 0$ illustrates the Wiener process with drift $\mu = 1$ and $\sigma = 8$ in the presence of an absorbing barrier at $a = 250$. The corresponding first-passage time density $g(t|a)$ shown in the upper part has a mean of 250. Shown in the lower part is the transition density $f(x, t|a)$ at time $t = 250$; it corresponds to a cross-section at $t = 250$ through $f(x, t|a)$ as shown in Fig. 4.1. The area under the transition density at time t (equal to 0.405 at $t = 250$) represents the probability of the process not to be absorbed up until t. It is therefore also equal to the area under the first-passage time density g above t, that is, to the right of the vertical line at $t = 250$

at x at time t when there is an absorbing barrier at a. For small t, the density will be narrowly concentrated around its start point and cover an area of 1, whereas for large t, it tends to zero for all x. This is because with increasing t, more and more paths, like the one shown in Fig. 4.2, will have reached the barrier at $x = a$ at some time in $[0, t]$ and be absorbed there. The area under the transition density from $-\infty$ to a at any time t represents the probability of the process *not* to be absorbed up until t. It is therefore also equal to the probability that the first-passage time $\mathbf{T}_a$ to a is larger than t. Thus, if we define as $G(t|a)$ the probability that $\mathbf{T}_a \le t$, then the basic relation between f and G is (Fig. 4.2)

$$1 - G(t|a) = \int_{-\infty}^{a} f(x, t|a)\, dx \tag{4.21}$$

Note that Eq. (4.21) represents the exact counterpart to the analogous relation for the simple random walk that we obtained in Exercise 6 of Chap. 2.

Given we know $f(x, t|a)$ from Eq. (4.20), we can now use this relation to determine the distribution function and the density of $\mathbf{T}_a$. Taking the negative derivative with respect to t in Eq. (4.21), we have

$$g(t|a) = -\int_{-\infty}^{a} \frac{\partial}{\partial t} f(x, t|a) \, dx$$

$$= -\frac{1}{2}\sigma^2 \int_{-\infty}^{a} \frac{\partial^2}{\partial x^2} f(x, t|a) \, dx + \mu \int_{-\infty}^{a} \frac{\partial}{\partial x} f(x, t|a) \, dx$$

because the transition density f obeys the forward Eq. (4.18). Carrying out the integration with respect to x, we have[2]

$$g(t|a) = -\frac{1}{2}\sigma^2 \frac{\partial}{\partial x} f(x, t|a) \Big|_{x=-\infty}^{x=a} + \mu f(x, t|a) \Big|_{x=-\infty}^{x=a}$$

The lower limits of both summands must vanish because the density $f(x, t|a)$ and its spatial derivative must tend to zero as $x \to -\infty$. We therefore have

$$g(t|a) = -\frac{1}{2}\sigma^2 \frac{\partial}{\partial x} f(x, t|a) \Big|_{x=a} + \mu f(x, t|a) \Big|_{x=a}$$

Next, we observe that the value of $f(x, t|a)$ evaluated at $x = a$ equals zero because of the boundary condition Eq. (4.19) for the absorbing barrier. This leaves us with the final result

$$g(t|a) = -\frac{1}{2}\sigma^2 \frac{\partial}{\partial x} f(x, t|a) \Big|_{x=a} = \frac{a}{\sigma\sqrt{2\pi t^3}} \exp\left[-\frac{(a - \mu t)^2}{2\sigma^2 t}\right] \quad (4.22)$$

Observe in Fig. 4.1 that at any t, the slope of f with respect to x near the absorbing barrier is negative. This is because the condition Eq. (4.19) forces $f = 0$ at the boundary, in combination with the fact that a density cannot be negative; thus f must decrease towards a. Comparing the left-hand side of Eq. (4.22) to Eq. (3.11), we see that $g(t|a)$ corresponds to the flux across $x = a$ in a drift-free diffusion process; this is because the additional flux component μf that appears in Eq. (4.13) is necessarily zero at $x = a$, due to the boundary condition at the barrier.

To focus on the aspects that are central to the derivation of $g(t|a)$, we have assumed that the Wiener process starts at $x_0 = 0$. What changes when the starting position is $x_0 \neq 0$? All critical considerations remain essentially the same because x_0 appears only as a constant in the forward Equation (4.18). That is, x_0 simply

---

[2] The generic symbol $f(x)|_{x=x_0}^{x=x_1}$ stands for $f(x_1) - f(x_0)$. In contrast, the symbol $f(x)|_{x=x_0}$ stands for "f evaluated at $x = x_0$", that is, for $f(x_0)$.

shifts the scale of the state space, and for general x_0, the solution corresponding to
Eq. (4.20) reads

$$f(x_0, x, t|a) = \frac{1}{\sigma\sqrt{2\pi t}} \left\{ \exp\left[-\frac{(x - x_0 - \mu t)^2}{2\sigma^2 t}\right] \right.$$

$$\left. - \exp\left(\frac{2\mu a}{\sigma^2}\right) \exp\left[-\frac{(x - x_0 - 2a - \mu t)^2}{2\sigma^2 t}\right] \right\} \qquad (4.23)$$

The same steps as before then lead to the formally more general version of the first-
passage time density

$$g(t|a, x_0) = \frac{a - x_0}{\sigma\sqrt{2\pi t^3}} \exp\left[-\frac{(a - x_0 - \mu t)^2}{2\sigma^2 t}\right] \qquad (4.24)$$

It is evident from the form of $g(t|a, x_0)$ that from the first-passage time alone, a and
x_0 are not separately identifiable, only the distance $a - x_0$ is. Similarly, all parameters
can without loss of generality always be re-scaled so that $\sigma = 1$. For example, the
first-passage time distribution of a Wiener process with $\mu = 10, \sigma = 5, a = 100$,
and $x_0 = 20$ is identical to that for $\mu = 2, \sigma = 1, a = 16$, and $x_0 = 0$. Given that
we can always transform g to an equivalent version with, say, $\sigma = 1$ and $x_0 = 0$,
the first-passage time distribution of a Wiener process in the presence of a single
absorbing barrier has in effect two unrelated parameters, the drift and the absorbing
barrier.

A simple but instructive thought experiment shows that the origin and scale of the
state space of a Wiener process is necessarily only fixed up to linear transformations.
Suppose A observes simulations such as the one shown in Fig. 4.2 of an original
Wiener process $X(t)$, characterized by some specific choice of $< \mu, \sigma, a, x_0 >$, the
barrier a represented as a horizontal line. Simultaneously, B observes projections of
these simulations onto a large screen. By elementary projective geometry, μ, σ, and
a as seen on the screen are then all scaled by the same magnifying factor, and the
origin on the projection screen is arbitrary. Yet, in any individual realization, A and
B will observe the first-passage to the absorbing line at exactly the same moment of
time and will therefore across many such simulations build up the same first-passage
time distribution.

Another assumption that we have made throughout so far is that the drift μ of the
Wiener process is positive, that is, directed toward the barrier, given a was assumed
to be above x_0. What changes in the analysis if the drift is away from the barrier,
that is, if $\mu < 0$ but $a > x_0$? All steps presented above actually remain valid even if
$\mu < 0$; for example, the forward Eq. (4.18) and also Eqs. (4.23) and (4.24) hold for
$\mu < 0$, too. What does change, though, is that for $\mu < 0$, the density Eq. (4.24) of
the first-passage time has a defect, that is, it does no longer integrate to 1 across t.
This means that there is then a finite probability that the Wiener process will never
reach the barrier at a.

Integrating the density g in Eq. (4.24) for $\mu < 0$, standard analysis results (e.g., Abramowitz and Stegun 1965, ch. 7.4) will show that this defect is equal to $1 - \exp[\frac{2\mu(a-x_0)}{\sigma^2}]$, representing the probability that $X(t)$ will never reach the barrier at a. If we divide the density Eq. (4.24) by the complementary probability $\exp[\frac{2\mu(a-x_0)}{\sigma^2}]$ of eventual absorption, then we obtain the *conditional* density of $\mathbf{T}_a$ given that the process ever reaches the barrier at a; this conditional density, g^* say, integrates to 1. As expected, these facts correspond closely to the situation for the simple random walk with a barrier at $a > 0$ when $p < \frac{1}{2}$; see Exercise 4 of Chap. 2.

In explicit form, carrying out this division, we then get for the case of $\mu < 0$ and $a > x_0$ the regular conditional density

$$g^*(t|a, x_0) = \frac{a - x_0}{\sigma\sqrt{2\pi t^3}} \exp\left[-\frac{(a - x_0 + \mu t)^2}{2\sigma^2 t}\right] \quad , \text{ for } \mu < 0 \quad (4.25)$$

This representation of g^* is remarkably similar to Eq. (4.24) for the case of $\mu > 0$ and permits us to write a general expression for the density (or conditional density, when $\mu < 0$) in the form of

$$\frac{a - x_0}{\sigma\sqrt{2\pi t^3}} \exp\left[-\frac{(a - x_0 - |\mu|t)^2}{2\sigma^2 t}\right] \quad (4.26)$$

If $\mu > 0$, then this is just the regular density Eq. (4.24), and if $\mu < 0$, then it is the conditional density given that absorption occurs, Eq. (4.25). Because only the absolute value of μ appears in Eq. (4.26), the result shows that this form is identical for two drift values μ differing only in sign. In this sense, then, we may say that for a negative drift, $X(t)$ will absorb at $a > x_0$ *less often*—that is, not always—but if it does absorb at all *not slower* than with the corresponding positive drift term.

4.2.2 The Backward Equation for First-Passage Times

The first-passage time density Eq. (4.24) is a basic result, and it is helpful to understand its direct relation not only to the forward Eq. (4.12) but also to the backward Eq. (4.16). To appreciate this relation, we consider in this section a second derivation of $g(t|a, x_0)$, based on the backward Eq. (4.16). As explained in Sect. 4.1.3, this equation relates changes of the time variable t to changes of the start point x_0, for a fixed value of the state (position) variable, x. As in many first-passage time problems the final (i.e., absorbing) state is fixed, the backward equation is often a natural choice in this context.

Consider a Wiener process $X(t)$ with drift $\mu > 0$ and variance σ^2 that starts at x_0, and assume that $a > x_0$ is an absorbing barrier. Let $F(x_0, x, t|a)$ denote the joint probability that:

 (i) during the interval $[0, t]$, the process never reached the level a
 (ii) at time t, the process is at or below some level x (where $x \le a$).

Clearly, F will also depend on μ and σ^2, but to keep our notation more parsimonious, and to focus on quantities considered variable in the following derivation, we suppress these constants for the moment.

By (i) and (ii), $F(x_0, x, t|a)$ is the integral of the transition density with respect to the position (state) variable, x. That is, we must have

$$F(x_0, x, t|a) = \int_{-\infty}^{x} f(x_0, v, t|a) \, dv \tag{4.27}$$

where f is the transition density Eq. (4.23) of the process, that is, the density to be at x at time t when the start is at x_0, and a is an absorbing barrier. As discussed in the previous section, when $a - x_0$ and μ have the same sign, then ultimate absorption at a is a certain event. Therefore, the function $F(x_0, x, t|a)$ must tend to zero as $t \to \infty$ because the condition (i) will ultimately not be satisfied.

As discussed in Sect. 4.2.1, at states below a, the local dynamics is not influenced by the presence of the barrier. For example, contemplating small changes of x_0 and t, the same local limiting operations as in Sect. 4.1.3 remain valid. Thus, even in the presence of a barrier at a, for $x < a$, the transition density f still satisfies the backward Eq. (4.16)

$$\frac{\partial f(x_0, x, t|a)}{\partial t} = \frac{1}{2}\sigma^2 \cdot \frac{\partial^2 f(x_0, x, t|a)}{\partial x_0^2} + \mu \cdot \frac{\partial f(x_0, x, t|a)}{\partial x_0}$$

As emphasized in Sect. 4.1.3, this equation relates changes in t to those in x_0, for a given spatial coordinate x. In view of the relation Eq. (4.27), integrating f across x, we see that F, too, satisfies the backward equation in t and x_0.

Furthermore, we note that for $x = a$, the condition (ii) above becomes redundant with condition (i), and thus the expression $F(x_0, a, t|a)$ simply refers to the probability (i) that during $[0, t]$, the process starting at x_0 never reached the level a. But this is the same as the event that the first passage to the level a takes place at some time later than t. That is, $F(x_0, a, t|a)$ simply represents the survivor function of the first-passage time $\mathbf{T}_a$,

$$F(x_0, a, t|a) = \mathsf{P}(\mathbf{T}_a > t) = 1 - G(t|a, x_0) \tag{4.28}$$

where $G(t|a, x_0)$ is the distribution function of the first-passage time $\mathbf{T}_a$ to the level a, starting from x_0.

Differentiating Eq. (4.28) with respect to t, we get for the corresponding density $g(t|a, x_0)$ of $\mathbf{T}_a$

$$g(t|a, x_0) = \frac{\partial[\mathsf{P}(\mathbf{T}_a \leq t)]}{\partial t} = -\frac{\partial[1 - G(t|a, x_0)]}{\partial t} = -\frac{\partial F(x_0, a, t|a)}{\partial t} \tag{4.29}$$

Now, we already know that F satisfies the backward Eq. (4.16). If F satisfies a linear differential equation such as Eq. (4.16), then the function $-\frac{\partial F(x_0, a, t|a)}{\partial t}$, that is, the density $g(t|a, x_0)$, must satisfy this equation, too. We thus get for the first-passage time density g the basic backward equation

$$\frac{\partial g(t|a, x_0)}{\partial t} = \frac{1}{2}\sigma^2 \cdot \frac{\partial^2 g(t|a, x_0)}{\partial x_0^2} + \mu \cdot \frac{\partial g(t|a, x_0)}{\partial x_0} \qquad (4.30)$$

It is tedious but not difficult in principle to show that $g(t|a, x_0)$ as given by Eq. (4.24) indeed satisfies Eq. (4.30).

4.2.3 An Alternative Derivation: The Moment-Generating Function

As stated in the previous two sections, the result Eq. (4.24) is basic, and so it is conceptually helpful to understand its direct relation to the discrete random walk discussed in Chap. 2. Thus, we next consider how the first-passage time density $g(t|a, x_0)$ may also be derived directly via the familiar limit operations based on the simple random walk model.

Consider a simple discrete random walk with step probability $p > \frac{1}{2}$ starting at 0. Based on an elementary first-step case distinction, we saw in Sect. 2.3.6 that the pgf $g(z)$ of the first-passage time $\mathbf{N}_1$ through the level $a = 1$ is

$$g(z) = \frac{1 - \sqrt{1 - 4p(1 - p)z^2}}{2(1 - p)z} \qquad (4.31)$$

We also explained in Sect. 2.3.6 that this implies that the pgf of the first-passage time $\mathbf{N}_m$ through the level m is given by $[g(z)]^m$.

We next ask: how can we translate Eq. (4.31) for discrete random walks into an equation about first-passage times for the Wiener process with drift? To this end, consider as we did before (Sect. 4.1.1) the more general case in which each step has duration Δt, and size $\pm \Delta x$, such that $p = \frac{1}{2}\left(1 + \frac{\mu}{\sigma}\sqrt{\Delta t}\right)$ and $\Delta x = \sigma\sqrt{\Delta t}$. Note that the assumption of $p > \frac{1}{2}$ translates into $\mu > 0$. As before, we are specifically interested in the passage to the continuous limit when the duration and size of each step tend to zero. In this analysis, we will neglect all powers of Δt higher than $\sqrt{\Delta t}$ (e.g., $\Delta t = (\sqrt{\Delta t})^2$) as in the limit of $\Delta t \to 0$ considered, these powers all vanish faster than $\sqrt{\Delta t}$.

The standard random walk implicitly assumes that $\Delta t = \Delta x = 1$. In the more general formulation, the $\mathbf{N}_m$ steps will lead the walk for the first time to the fixed level $a = m \Delta x$, so that $m = \frac{a}{\Delta x}$. Also, in the more general formulation, the time needed to get to the level a for the first time is $\mathbf{T}_a = \mathbf{N}_m \Delta t = \mathbf{N}_{\frac{a}{\Delta x}} \Delta t$. Finally, we replace $z = e^{-s}$, that is, we go from a pgf for the discrete random variable $\mathbf{N}_m$ to an mgf for the continuous random variable $\mathbf{T}_a$. We then obtain the basic relation for the mgf of $\mathbf{T}_a$

$$m(s|a) = \mathrm{E}[\exp(-s\mathbf{T}_a)] = \mathrm{E}[\exp(-s\,\mathbf{N}_{\frac{a}{\Delta x}}\,\Delta t)] = [g(e^{-s\Delta t})]^{\frac{a}{\Delta x}} \qquad (4.32)$$

where g is the pgf of $\mathbf{N}_1$ as given in Eq. (4.31), and we have used the fact that the pgf of $\mathbf{N}_{\frac{a}{\Delta x}}$ is $[g(z)]^{a/\Delta x}$. Explicitly, then,

$$m(s|a) = \lim_{\substack{\Delta t \to 0 \\ \Delta x \to 0}} \left[\frac{1 - \sqrt{1 - 4p(1-p)e^{-2s\Delta t}}}{2(1-p)e^{-s\Delta t}} \right]^{\frac{a}{\Delta x}} \qquad (4.33)$$

Figure 4.3 illustrates that the right-hand side of Eq. (4.33) is an excellent approximation to $m(s|a)$, even when the discretization is relatively coarse, that is, when Δt is not small relative to the mean of $\mathbf{T}_a$. To determine the indicated limits, we next consider the numerator and denominator of $m(s|a)$ separately (e.g., Stewart 2012, ch. 1.6).

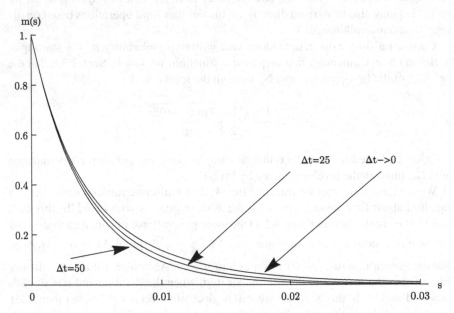

Fig. 4.3 The graph shows the right-hand side of Eq. (4.33) for $\mu = 1, \sigma = 8, a = 250$, for step durations of $\Delta t = 50$ (lowest curve) and $\Delta t = 25$ (middle), using $\Delta x = \sigma\sqrt{\Delta t}$, and the relation $p = \frac{1}{2}\left(1 + \frac{\mu}{\sigma}\sqrt{\Delta t}\right)$. Ordinate, moment-generating function $m(s)$; abscissa, s, the argument of m. The limiting top curve is the mgf $m(s)$ of the first-passage time $\mathbf{T}_a$ as given by Eq. (4.34). For these values, the mean first-passage time is 250, so that step durations of $\Delta t = 50$ represent a fairly coarse discretization. For $\Delta t = 1$, the difference between the true mgf $m(s)$ and the approximation based on the discrete simple random walk would not be discernable on the scale of the figure

Considering the numerator, the relation $p = \frac{1}{2}\left(1 + \frac{\mu}{\sigma}\sqrt{\Delta t}\right)$ implies that $4p(1 - p) = 1 - \left(\frac{\mu}{\sigma}\right)^2 \Delta t$. Also, for small Δt, we have $\exp(-2s\Delta t) \approx 1 - 2s\Delta t$. Together, then, ignoring powers higher than $\sqrt{\Delta t}$

$$1 - \sqrt{1 - 4p(1 - p)e^{-2s\Delta t}} \approx 1 - \frac{\sqrt{\Delta t}}{\sigma}\sqrt{2s\sigma^2 + \mu^2}$$

We next write the exponent in Eq. (4.33) in the form of $\frac{a}{\Delta x} = \frac{a}{\sigma\sqrt{\Delta t}} = w$ so that $\sqrt{\Delta t} = \frac{a}{\sigma w}$; in terms of w, the numerator in Eq. (4.33) then tends to

$$\left[1 - \frac{a}{w\sigma^2}\sqrt{2s\sigma^2 + \mu^2}\right]^w$$

For $\Delta t \to 0$, we have $w \to \infty$, and the limit of the numerator in Eq. (4.33) takes the familiar form of $\lim_{w\to\infty}(1 - \frac{c}{w})^w = \exp(-c)$, with $c = \frac{a}{\sigma^2}\sqrt{2s\sigma^2 + \mu^2}$.

The limit for the denominator in Eq. (4.33) is found similarly, but simpler. For small Δt,

$$2(1 - p)e^{-s\Delta t} \approx \left(1 - \frac{\mu}{\sigma}\sqrt{\Delta t}\right)(1 - s\Delta t)$$

$$\approx 1 - \frac{\mu}{\sigma}\sqrt{\Delta t}$$

as all powers of Δt higher than $\sqrt{\Delta t}$ vanish as $\Delta t \to 0$. Again writing the exponent in the form $\frac{a}{\Delta x} = \frac{a}{\sigma\sqrt{\Delta t}} = w$, we see that the denominator in Eq. (4.33) tends to

$$\left(1 - \frac{a\mu}{w\sigma^2}\right)^w$$

which is again of the form $\lim_{w\to\infty}(1 - \frac{c}{w})^w = \exp(-c)$, now with $c = \frac{a\mu}{\sigma^2}$.

Dividing the independent limits of the numerator and denominator in Eq. (4.33), we finally get for $a > 0$

$$m(s|a) = \mathsf{E}[\exp(-s\mathbf{T}_a)] = \exp\left[\frac{a}{\sigma^2}\left(\mu - \sqrt{2s\sigma^2 + \mu^2}\right)\right] \qquad (4.34)$$

for the mgf of the first-passage time $\mathbf{T}_a$. As discussed in the previous section, if the start is at $x_0 < a$ rather than at 0, then we would need to replace a by $a - x_0$.

Given that there is a one-to-one relation between a density and its mgf, $g(t|a, x_0)$ is in principle given by $m(s|a)$. At least in hindsight, it is straightforward (if tedious) to verify that in fact

$$m(s|a) = \int_0^\infty e^{-st} g(t|a, x_0)\, dt$$

with g given in Eq. (4.22). The basic insight from this derivation, though, is that the first-passage time problem for the Wiener process can be directly understood, and analyzed, in terms of the simple random walk whose discrete nature is conceptually readily accessible and, for example, easily simulated.

We can use this conceptual analogy to further illustrate the nature of the limiting process leading to Eq. (4.34). Consider again the case of $\mu = 1, \sigma = 8$, and $a = 250$ that is also illustrated in Figs. 4.1 and 4.2. For these values, the mean first-passage time of the Wiener process to the barrier at $a = 250$ is equal to 250 (see Exercise 4). Choosing $\Delta t = 50$ will then evidently represent a fairly coarse discretization compared to the mean first-passage time. The random walk then has steps of absolute size $\Delta x = \sigma \sqrt{\Delta t} = 56.6$, and the step probability is $p = \frac{1}{2}\left(1 + \frac{\mu}{\sigma}\sqrt{\Delta t}\right) = 0.942$. When the barrier at $a = 250$ is scaled in step size units, it equals $a/\Delta x = 4.42$. In effect, this means that we compare the original Wiener process to a discrete random walk in which each step takes 50 time units, with step sizes of 1 and a barrier at 4.42. We know from Eq. (2.18) that it will take this discrete random walk on average $4.42/(2 \cdot 0.942 - 1) = 5$ steps to cross the barrier at 4.42. When each of these steps takes 50 time units, then the mean first-passage time will be 250 for the discrete random walk as well. With the standard relations used in the limiting process above, it is straightforward to show that this equivalence in means holds generally.

4.3   One Reflecting Barrier

In many diffusion contexts, a natural question to ask is: When does the process first reach some particular position? As we have seen, this type of question leads to the concept of absorbing barriers—the intuitive physical notion being that a particle approaching this type of barrier gets permanently stuck there. An alternative form of barrier in diffusion is based on the notion that a particle reaching it is *reflected* rather than being absorbed by it.

A simple real-world analogy for a process with a reflecting barrier is a fly that either moves away from a windowpane or else bumps into it, but can never traverse it. Another example is the temperature of water that (under normal pressure) can approach but never exceed 100 °C. A more formal discrete analogy is a simple random walk that upon reaching the reflecting barrier in the next step moves with probability p one step away from it or with probability $1 - p$ remains at that barrier, as it cannot move on beyond it. In this scenario, the local dynamics at all other states further away from the reflecting barrier (recall the derivation via a discrete random walk in Sect. 4.1.1) remains just the same as before.

4.3.1 Reflecting Barrier in the Absence of Drift

To emphasize the main conceptual points, let us begin with the simplest case. That is, consider a drift-free diffusion process $\{X(t), t \geq 0\}$, with variance parameter σ^2 starting at a position $X(0) = x_0 > a$; however, its free diffusive evolution is delimited by a reflecting barrier placed below x_0 at $x = a$. In the absence of an additional absorbing barrier, the main interest focuses on the transition density f for $X(t)$ to be at a particular position x at time $t > 0$. Relative to free diffusion, the presence of a reflecting barrier will evidently modify the transition density; for example, f must integrate to 1 across all states $x \geq a$. To make this dependence explicit, we write $f(x, t|a)$ for the density of the process to be at x at time t when a reflecting barrier is placed at $x = a$, where it is understood that f also depends on $x_0 > a$ and σ^2.

Note that relative to free, unconstrained diffusion, a reflecting barrier at $x = a$ will tend to *increase* f for $x > a$ because now the particle cannot escape to the left of (or below) the reflecting boundary at $x = a$. But how large exactly is this "increase"? The answer can be found by an elegant argument, the reflection principle (e.g., Takacs 1986).

Consider first a particle moving in a free diffusion process with zero drift starting at x_0, that is, without a reflecting barrier at $x = a$. We know from Sect. 3.2.1 that at time t, its position will be normally distributed, with mean x_0 and variance $\sigma^2 t$. As shown in the upper part of Fig. 4.4, without altering the diffusive movement itself, we may imagine to bend the $x-$axis along which this particle moves at the point $x = a$, such that the point $a - z$ lies just below the point $a + z$ (i.e., the sum of both coordinates is $2a$).

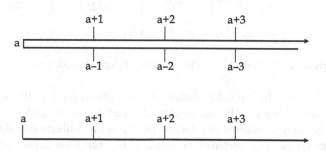

spatial position of the particle

Fig. 4.4 Upper panel: A particle moves in a regular free diffusion process, but the axis along which it moves is sharply bent at $x = a$, so that for $x < a$, the point $a - z$ lies just below the point $a + z$. Lower panel: A second particle moves on the half-line $[a, \infty)$ such that its position is $a + z$ if and only if the position of the first particle is either $a + z$ or $a - z$. Thus, the second particle's position is given by the perpendicular projection of the position of the first particle: locally, it moves as in a regular diffusion process, but with a built-in reflecting barrier placed at $x = a$. We assume the bend (the short vertical line at $x = a$ in the upper panel) to be of negligible length

Next, consider a second particle moving on the half-line $[a, \infty)$ such that its position is $a + z$ if and only if the position of the first particle is either $a + z$ or $a - z$. Thus, the second particle (lower panel) moves like the perpendicular projection of the position of the first particle (upper panel). Clearly, the second particle then also moves as in a regular diffusion process, but with a built-in reflecting barrier placed at $x = a$. At time t, it will occupy the position x if and only if at time t the first particle, in the free diffusion process, occupies either position x or position $2a - x$ (the sum of both coordinates being $2a$); these events are mutually exclusive so that their densities add.

Observe that this argument requires displacements of the same size to the left and right to be equally probable; for example, a displacement from $a - 2$ down to $a - 3$ in the upper panel of Fig. 4.4 corresponds to a displacement from $a + 2$ up to $a + 3$ in the lower panel of Fig. 4.4.

We know from Eq. (3.8) that the position of the first particle (free diffusion) after time t has a normal density with mean x_0 and variance $\sigma^2 t$. Therefore, the argument illustrated in Fig. 4.4 gives for the second particle moving in the presence of a reflecting barrier at $x = a$ the transition density

$$f(x, t | a) = \frac{1}{\sigma\sqrt{2\pi t}} \exp\left[-\frac{(x - x_0)^2}{2\sigma^2 t}\right] + \frac{1}{\sigma\sqrt{2\pi t}} \exp\left[-\frac{(2a - x - x_0)^2}{2\sigma^2 t}\right] \quad (4.35)$$

for $x \geq a$. Clearly, all that matters here is the distance of the starting point x_0 to the reflecting barrier at a, which, therefore, we may place at $a = 0$ without loss of generality. This gives the slightly more compact result

$$f(x, t | a = 0) = \frac{1}{\sigma\sqrt{2\pi t}} \exp\left[-\frac{(x - x_0)^2}{2\sigma^2 t}\right] + \frac{1}{\sigma\sqrt{2\pi t}} \exp\left[-\frac{(-x - x_0)^2}{2\sigma^2 t}\right]$$

$$= n(x | x_0, \sigma^2 t) + n(-x | x_0, \sigma^2 t) \quad (4.36)$$

for $x \geq 0$, where as usual $n(x | \mu, \sigma^2)$ is the normal density with mean μ and variance σ^2.

Figure 4.5 shows the typical evolution of f with time, for $\sigma = 10$, $x_0 = 200$, and a reflecting barrier at $a = 0$. For a short initial time interval, the process is typically still narrowly confined around the starting point, and no influence of the reflecting barrier is yet visible. For intermediate values t, the transition density still shows a clear mode which moves slowly from x_0 toward 0; however, the mass in the region close to the barrier is now staunched, as there can be no flux across $a = 0$. Finally, for large t, the density simply falls off with the distance to the reflecting barrier.

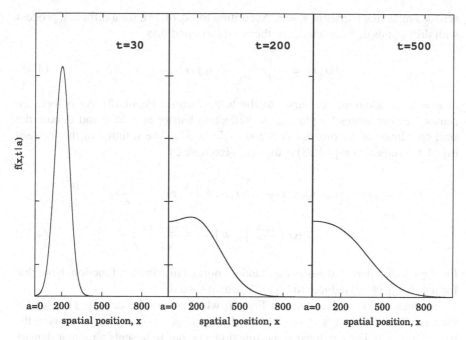

Fig. 4.5 Three transition densities $f(x, t|a)$ (ordinate) for $\sigma = 10$, $x_0 = 200$, and a reflecting barrier at $a = 0$, as shown on the abscissa. Left panel refers to $t = 30$ when the process is typically still close to its starting point $x_0 = 200$. Middle panel for $t = 200$ shows the staunching effect of the reflecting barrier at $a = 0$ on $f(x, t|a)$. Right panel: for large $t = 500$, the density $f(x, t|a)$ falls off with increasing distance from the barrier. Note that for all t, the density f approaches the barrier horizontally from the right, which means that the slope of f vanishes close to the reflecting barrier

4.3.2   Reflecting Barrier in the Presence of Drift

We may verify from the general result Eq. (4.35) that the local density gradient at the reflecting barrier $x = a$ is

$$\left. \frac{\partial f}{\partial x} \right|_{x=a} = 0 \tag{4.37}$$

We have seen in Chap. 3 (cf., Eq. (3.11)) that the flux in a drift-free unrestricted diffusion process across a coordinate $x = a$ at time t is generally equal to $J(a, t) = -\frac{1}{2}\sigma^2 \frac{\partial f}{\partial x}\big|_{x=a}$. Therefore, Eq. (4.37) formalizes the intuitive notion that due to the reflecting effect of the barrier, the probability flux $J(a, t)$ across the barrier equals zero. In Fig. 4.5, this feature is indicated by the horizontal approach of f from the right to the boundary at $a = 0$.

We can use these observations for the definition of a reflecting barrier a in more general diffusion processes, which is based on the notion of zero flux of probability across a reflecting barrier at $x = a$. According to Eq. (4.13), for a diffusion process with drift μ, this definition leads to the boundary condition

$$J(x, t) = -\frac{1}{2}\sigma^2\frac{\partial f}{\partial x} + \mu\, f(x, t|a) = 0 \tag{4.38}$$

at $x = a$, in addition, of course, to the basic forward Eq. (4.12). As before, we center the coordinates by placing the reflecting barrier at $a = 0$ and denote the start coordinate of the process as $X(t = 0) = x_0 > a$. The solution of the forward Eq. (4.12) subject to Eq. (4.38) is then (cf., Exercise 2)

$$f(x, t|a = 0) = \left[n(x|x_0, \sigma^2 t) + n(-x|x_0, \sigma^2 t)\right] \cdot \exp\left[\frac{\mu(x - x_0)}{\sigma^2} - \frac{\mu^2 t}{2\sigma^2}\right]$$

$$- \frac{2\mu}{\sigma^2} \cdot \exp\left(\frac{2\mu x}{\sigma^2}\right) \cdot \Phi\left(-\frac{x + x_0 + \mu t}{\sigma\sqrt{t}}\right) \tag{4.39}$$

for $x \geq a = 0$, where Φ denotes the standard normal distribution function. Note that for $\mu = 0$, Eq. (4.39) reduces to Eq. (4.36), as it should.

Equation (4.39) is illustrated in Fig. 4.6 which shows the density $f(x, t|a)$ for the case when the start is at $x_0 = 100$ and the drift $\mu = -1$ is directed toward the barrier at $a = 0$. For any fixed t, the function $f(x, t|a)$ represents a regular density across the state variable x. Thus, we can cut a slice through $f(x, t|a)$ at various time points $t = 10, 30, 100$ to illustrate the typical evolution of this process in more detail. These slices are shown in Fig. 4.7. Initially, the diffusion process is still narrowly confined around its starting point x_0. If x_0 is sufficiently distant from the barrier a, then no influence of the barrier is yet seen at this stage. For intermediate values of t, the transition density exhibits more complex dynamics: due to the negative drift, the main mode keeps traveling toward the barrier, but between this mode and the barrier, there develops a low point. It reflects the tailback of the diffusion at the barrier, as there is no flux across $a = 0$. For large t, the low point disappears and gives way to a monotone decline of the density as the distance to the reflecting barrier increases.

Note that in contrast to the drift-free case shown in Fig. 4.5, the slope of the density at the barrier $a = 0$ in Fig. 4.7 is no longer zero, as is expected from the boundary condition Eq. (4.38). Geometrically, this boundary condition means that the slope of f at $a = 0$ equals $\frac{2\mu}{\sigma^2} f$, that is, it is proportional to f itself. When the process drifts toward the barrier (so that $\mu < 0$), then the constant of proportionality $\frac{2\mu}{\sigma^2}$ is negative. This indicates that the decline of f at $x = 0$ gets steeper as f increases, that is, as the reflecting barrier staunches the density at $x = 0$.

The final stage shown in Fig. 4.7 refers to the limiting density to which Eq. (4.39) converges when the drift is directed toward the reflecting barrier. It is instructive to obtain this density by considering the forward Eq. (4.12) when the derivative of f with respect to the time variable vanishes:

$$\frac{\partial f}{\partial t} = \frac{1}{2}\sigma^2\frac{\partial^2 f}{\partial x^2} - \mu\frac{\partial f}{\partial x} = 0 \tag{4.40}$$

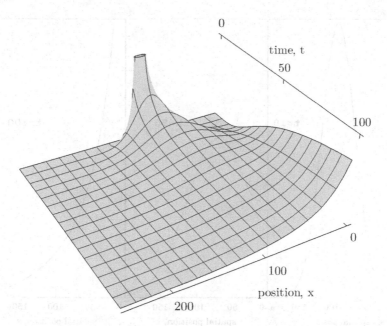

Fig. 4.6 The evolution of the transition density $f(x, t|a)$ as given by Eq. (4.39) of a Wiener process starting at $x_0 = 100$ in the presence of a reflecting barrier at $a = 0$, for $\mu = -1, \sigma = 8$. Right axis, time t; front axis, spatial position x of the process; vertical axis, density $f(x, t|a)$; the reflecting barrier a is placed at the spatial coordinate $x = 0$. For small t, the density f is narrowly confined around the starting point at $x_0 = 100$; for intermediate t, the staunching effect of the reflecting barrier produces a low point between the mode and the reflecting barrier at $a = 0$; for large t, the density decreases with the distance from the barrier

Equation (4.40) is an ordinary first-order differential equation for the function $\frac{\partial f}{\partial x}$. When the drift is toward the reflecting barrier ($\mu < 0$), the solution is a regular exponential density $f(x, \infty|a = 0) = \lambda \exp(-\lambda x)$ with rate $\lambda = -\frac{2\mu}{\sigma^2} > 0$. When the drift is away from the reflecting barrier ($\mu > 0$), the process will spread out more and more across the interval $[0, \infty]$, and no limiting density exists.

The limiting exponential density for $\mu < 0$ represents a compromise, or an equilibrium, between the purely diffusive process on the one hand, leading to dissipation along the positive line, and the negative drift term on the other which serves to drive the process to pile up at the reflecting barrier. It is readily confirmed that the solution $f(x, \infty|a = 0)$ corresponds to the limit of Eq. (4.39) for $t \to \infty$, as it must. These results imply that, independent of x_0, for $\mu < 0$ and $a = 0$, the mean and standard deviation of $X(t)$ tend to $-\frac{\sigma^2}{2\mu}$ for large t; for the example shown in Fig. 4.7, this limit equals 32. Note that the limiting exponential density $f(x, \infty|a = 0)$ still satisfies the boundary condition Eq. (4.38).

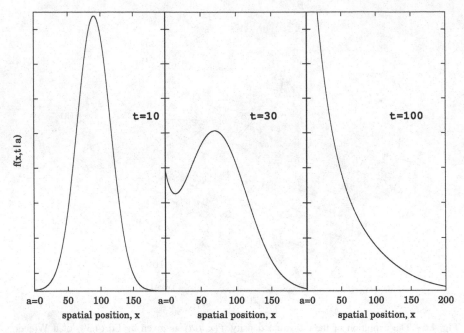

Fig. 4.7   Three transition densities $f(x, t|a)$ (ordinate) for $\mu = -1, \sigma = 8, x_0 = 100$, and a reflecting barrier at $a = 0$, as shown on the abscissa; compare to Fig. 4.6. Left panel refers to $t = 10$ when the process is typically still close to its starting point $x_0 = 100$. Middle panel for $t = 30$ shows the complex staunching effect on $f(x, t|a)$, with a low point between the mode and the reflecting barrier at $a = 0$. Right panel: for large $t = 100$, the density $f(x, t|a)$ falls off exponentially with increasing distance to the barrier

4.4   Two Absorbing Barriers

When the Wiener process is confined by two barriers, the scenario involving two *absorbing* barriers is most relevant in applications. Therefore, we will consider this case in some detail, including explicit computational aspects. The remaining cases of two reflecting barriers and the mixed case are clearly less prominent in applications. Correspondingly, it is treated here in less detail.

As we have already seen in Chap. 2, in the context of the discrete random walk, when there are two absorbing barriers, then several new aspects need to be addressed which are not present in the case of a single barrier. For example, the process may absorb at either barrier, and we are interested to know what is the probability to absorb at the upper rather than at the lower barrier. Related to this distinction, we may consider properties of the first-passage time, such as its distribution or its mean, conditional on absorbing at the upper (or at the lower) barrier. In the following sections, we first look at absorption probabilities and the (conditional) mean first-passage times and then at the full distribution of the first-passage times.

4.4.1 Absorption Probability

Following our reasoning in Sect. 4.1.1, a straightforward approach is to interpret the Wiener process as a limit of the simple random walk in which each step has duration Δt and size $\pm \Delta x$, such that $\Delta x = \sigma \sqrt{\Delta t}$ and $p = \frac{1}{2}\left(1 + \frac{\mu}{\sigma}\sqrt{\Delta t}\right)$, or with p expressed in terms of Δx, $p = \frac{1}{2}\left(1 + \frac{\mu}{\sigma^2}\Delta x\right)$. The latter relation indicates that the sign of μ then corresponds to whether in the corresponding random walk, p is smaller or larger than $\frac{1}{2}$. As before, we are specifically interested in the passage to the continuous limit when the duration and size of each step tend to zero. Note that as far as the absorption probability is concerned, the temporal scale of the process is in effect irrelevant.

The standard simple random walk implicitly assumes that $\Delta t = \Delta x = 1$. Correspondingly, in the more general formulation, the distance of the barriers from the starting point is measured in multiples of the size of each individual step, that is, as $\frac{a}{\Delta x}$ and $\frac{b}{\Delta x}$. In fact, we already used this relation in Sect. 4.2.3 to derive the mgf of the first-passage time for the Wiener process in the case of a single absorbing barrier. For example, when $\Delta x = 0.1$, then barriers placed at ± 5 correspond to a standard simple random walk with barriers placed at ± 50.

In Chap. 2, we saw (cf., Eq. (2.13)) that for a standard simple random walk starting at zero, the probability to absorb at a rather than at $-b$ equals

$$\psi(p|a, b) = \frac{1 - \eta^b}{1 - \eta^{a+b}} \tag{4.41}$$

where $\eta = \frac{1-p}{p}$. Inserting now into the definition of η the relation $p = \frac{1}{2}\left(1 + \frac{\mu}{\sigma^2}\Delta x\right)$, we have

$$\eta(\Delta x) = \frac{1 - \frac{\mu}{\sigma^2}\Delta x}{1 + \frac{\mu}{\sigma^2}\Delta x} \tag{4.42}$$

and from Eq. (4.41), the absorption probability we are looking for is the limit

$$\psi(\mu, \sigma^2|a, b) = \lim_{\Delta x \to 0} \frac{1 - [\eta(\Delta x)]^{b/\Delta x}}{1 - [\eta(\Delta x)]^{(a+b)/\Delta x}} \tag{4.43}$$

We first determine the limit of the expression $\eta^{1/\Delta x}$ that appears in both the numerator and the denominator of Eq. (4.43), rewriting this expression from the definition of η in Eq. (4.42) in the form of

$$\lim_{\Delta x \to 0} [\eta(\Delta x)]^{1/\Delta x} = \lim_{\Delta x \to 0} \frac{\left[1 - \frac{\mu/\sigma^2}{1/\Delta x}\right]^{1/\Delta x}}{\left[1 + \frac{\mu/\sigma^2}{1/\Delta x}\right]^{1/\Delta x}}$$

We see that both the numerator and the denominator are of the familiar general form $\lim_{m \to \infty} \left(1 + \frac{\alpha}{m}\right)^m = e^\alpha$, and so we obtain

$$\lim_{\Delta x \to 0} [\eta(\Delta x)]^{1/\Delta x} = \frac{\exp\left(-\frac{\mu}{\sigma^2}\right)}{\exp\left(+\frac{\mu}{\sigma^2}\right)} = \exp\left(-\frac{2\mu}{\sigma^2}\right)$$

We next insert this limit separately into the numerator and denominator of Eq. (4.43) to get the probability to absorb at a

$$p_a = \psi(\mu, \sigma^2 | a, b) = \frac{1 - \exp\left(-\frac{2\mu b}{\sigma^2}\right)}{1 - \exp\left(-\frac{2\mu(a+b)}{\sigma^2}\right)} \tag{4.44}$$

4.4.2 Mean First-Passage Times

Conceptually, the limiting procedure for the conditional mean first-passage times proceeds along lines very similar to our approach in Sect. 4.4.1. In Chap. 2, we have seen (Eq. (2.26)) that for a standard simple random walk starting at zero, the conditional mean number of steps, given the walk absorbs at barrier a, is equal to

$$E_a[N] = \frac{1}{2p - 1} \cdot \left\{ (a + b) \frac{1 + \eta^{a+b}}{1 - \eta^{a+b}} - b \frac{1 + \eta^b}{1 - \eta^b} \right\} \tag{4.45}$$

When each step is of size $\pm \Delta x$ and takes Δt time units, then the distance to the barriers is scaled in units Δx, and the real time to absorption is the number of steps, multiplied by Δt, the time per step. We therefore need to inspect the limit

$$\lim_{\Delta x \to 0, \Delta t \to 0} \frac{\Delta t}{2p - 1} \cdot \left\{ \frac{a + b}{\Delta x} \frac{1 + [\eta(\Delta x)]^{(a+b)/\Delta x}}{1 - [\eta(\Delta x)]^{(a+b)/\Delta x}} - \frac{b}{\Delta x} \frac{1 + [\eta(\Delta x)]^{b/\Delta x}}{1 - [\eta(\Delta x)]^{b/\Delta x}} \right\}$$

To this end, it is easiest to look first at the generic limit expression

$$\lim_{\Delta x \to 0, \Delta t \to 0} \frac{\Delta t}{2p - 1} \cdot \frac{c}{\Delta x} \frac{1 + [\eta(\Delta x)]^{c/\Delta x}}{1 - [\eta(\Delta x)]^{c/\Delta x}}$$

then setting $c = a + b$, $c = b$ in turn. We insert the relations $2p - 1 = (\mu/\sigma^2)\Delta x$ and $\Delta t = (\Delta x)^2/\sigma^2$ to get

$$\lim_{\Delta x \to 0, \Delta t \to 0} \frac{(\Delta x)^2/\sigma^2}{(\mu/\sigma^2)\Delta x} \cdot \frac{c}{\Delta x} \frac{1 + [\eta(\Delta x)]^{c/\Delta x}}{1 - [\eta(\Delta x)]^{c/\Delta x}} = \frac{c}{\mu} \frac{1 + \exp\left(-\frac{2\mu c}{\sigma^2}\right)}{1 - \exp\left(-\frac{2\mu c}{\sigma^2}\right)}$$

using the limit of $[\eta(\Delta x)]^{1/\Delta x}$ that we had already determined in Sect. 4.4.1 to find the absorption probabilities. Inserting $c = a + b, c = b$ into this result, we obtain for the mean conditional first-passage time

$$E_a[T] = \frac{1}{\mu} \left[(a + b) \frac{1 + \exp\left(-\frac{2\mu(a+b)}{\sigma^2}\right)}{1 - \exp\left(-\frac{2\mu(a+b)}{\sigma^2}\right)} - b \frac{1 + \exp\left(-\frac{2\mu b}{\sigma^2}\right)}{1 - \exp\left(-\frac{2\mu b}{\sigma^2}\right)} \right] \tag{4.46}$$

The corresponding result for $E_{-b}[T]$ can be obtained by interchanging a and b and using $\mu' = -\mu$. Slight algebraic rearrangements then give

$$E_{-b}[T] = \frac{1}{\mu} \left[(a + b) \frac{1 + \exp\left(-\frac{2\mu(a+b)}{\sigma^2}\right)}{1 - \exp\left(-\frac{2\mu(a+b)}{\sigma^2}\right)} - a \frac{1 + \exp\left(-\frac{2\mu a}{\sigma^2}\right)}{1 - \exp\left(-\frac{2\mu a}{\sigma^2}\right)} \right] \tag{4.47}$$

As we discussed in Sect. 2.3.5, a more comprehensible version of these unwieldy results is

$$E_a[T] = h(a + b) - h(b) \tag{4.48}$$

where $h(t) = (t/\mu) \coth(\mu t/\sigma^2)$. Similarly,

$$E_{-b}[T] = h(a + b) - h(a) \tag{4.49}$$

Clearly, $E_a[T]$ and $E_{-b}[T]$ exhibit the same properties as those discussed in detail in Sect. 2.3.5 and shown in Fig. 2.9. The similarity of Eqs. (4.46) and (4.47) to Eq. (2.26) seems striking at first, but essentially it reflects the close conceptual correspondence in the construction of both processes. Seen in this light, the Wiener process may appear as a mere notational variant of the simple random walk, mediated by the central limit theorem. However, the concepts that we use to analyze it can be translated to more general processes, several of which will be described in Chaps. 5 and 6.

It is another remarkable feature of Eqs. (4.46) and (4.47) that changing the sign of the drift rate has no effect at all on either $E_a[T]$ or $E_{-b}[T]$. This is seen from the fact that the function h in Eqs. (4.48) and (4.49) is symmetric with respect to the drift: $h(t|\mu) = h(t| - \mu)$. Therefore, replacing μ with $-\mu$ influences the probability to absorb at a (as given by Eq. (4.44)), but it does not alter the mean time to reach it.

Of course, the overall mean first-passage time is the mean of $E_a[T]$ and $E_{-b}[T]$, weighted by the respective absorption probabilities. Using the results in Eqs. 4.44, 4.46, and 4.47, we find that

$$E[T] = \frac{a \, p_a - b \, p_{-b}}{\mu} \tag{4.50}$$

As discussed for discrete random walks in Sect. 2.3.4, this expression can be interpreted as the mean position at the moment of absorption (which is either a or $-b$), divided by the mean displacement (equal to μ) per time unit.

4.4.3 First-Passage Time Distributions

Conceptually, many aspects of the analysis of first-passage time distributions carry over from the simpler case of a single absorbing barrier, considered in Sect. 4.2.1. Specifically, the transition density $f(x, t|a, b)$ in the presence of absorbing barriers at a and $-b$ is the basic quantity, and the first-passage time densities follow by a direct relation to f that is based on a consideration of the probability flux across the barriers. For a given starting state, such as $x_0 = 0$, the transition density f still satisfies the forward Equation (4.18) in the state variable x and the time variable t. Also, the initial condition is again such that for $t \to 0$, the density f must be concentrated at x_0; if not mentioned otherwise, for the rest of this chapter, we assume that $x_0 = 0$. However, corresponding to Eq. (4.19), there are now two boundary conditions that must be fulfilled by f at all t,

$$f(-b, t|a, b) = f(a, t|a, b) = 0 \qquad \text{for } t > 0 \tag{4.51}$$

Also, we now have two separate first-passage time densities, one referring to absorptions at the upper barrier a and one referring to absorptions at the lower barrier $-b$. To distinguish them, we denote them as $g_+(t|a, b)$ and $g_-(t|a, b)$, respectively, where it is understood that g_+ and g_- also depend on μ and σ^2; the corresponding distribution functions are denoted as G_+ and G_-.

It is essential to understand the conceptual meaning of these functions. The relation of f to g_+ and g_- is illustrated in Fig. 4.8, which corresponds to Fig. 4.2 for the case of a single absorbing barrier. The area under the transition density f at any time t again represents the probability of the process not to be absorbed up until t. It is therefore also equal to the sum of the areas under the first-passage time densities g_+ and g_- above t. As $t \to \infty$, this implies that the overall probability to absorb (at any time) at the upper barrier a is equal to the total area under g_+. Similarly, the area under g_- corresponds to the overall probability to absorb (at any time) at the lower barrier $-b$.

If we write more formally $\mathbf{T}_{ab}$ for the first-passage time between the barriers $-b$ and a, then $X(\mathbf{T}_{ab})$ denotes the position of the Wiener process at the moment of its absorption, which must be either a or $-b$. Thus, we also have that $p_a = P[X(\mathbf{T}_{ab}) = a]$ is the probability to absorb at a, as given by Eq. (4.44). In this notation, the *joint* density g_+ is formally defined in terms of $\mathbf{T}_{ab}$ as $g_+(t|a, b) = P[\mathbf{T}_{ab} = t, X(\mathbf{T}_{ab}) = a]$. By elementary probability, the *conditional* density $P[\mathbf{T}_{ab} = t|X(\mathbf{T}_{ab}) = a]$ is then given by $g_+(t|a, b)/p_a$. For example, the conditional mean first-passage times derived in Sect. 4.4.2 refer to the mean of these conditional (or normalized) densities, that is, formally to, for example, $\int_0^\infty t\, g_+(t|a, b)dt/p_a$.

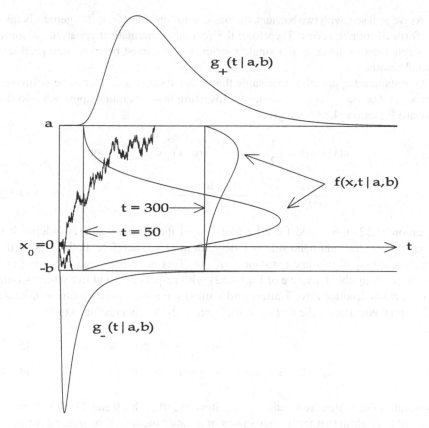

Fig. 4.8 The relation of the transition density $f(x, t|a, b)$ to the first-passage time densities $g_+(t|a, b)$ (shown at the top) and $g_-(t|a, b)$ (bottom); the abscissa represents time (t) and the ordinate the spatial position (x), including the barriers at $-b$ and a and the starting point at $x_0 = 0$. Two sample paths starting at $x_0 = 0$ illustrate the Wiener process with drift $\mu = 1$ and $\sigma = 8$ in the presence of absorbing barriers at $a = 250$ and $-b = -50$. Shown in the central part is the transition density $f(x, t|a, b)$ at times $t = 50$ and $t = 300$. The area under the transition density at time t represents the probability of the process not to be absorbed up until t. It is therefore also equal to the sum of the areas under the first-passage time densities g_+ and g_- above t. At $t = 50$, only few paths (a proportion of 0.143) have yet reached any barrier. Those that have are nearly all absorbed at the lower barrier that is closer to the starting point. At $t = 300$, the bulk (a proportion of 0.847) of all paths has been absorbed. As indicated by the areas under g_+ and g_-, at this point, clearly more paths (0.639) are absorbed at the upper than at the lower barrier (0.208). The area under f represents the small remaining proportion (0.153) that has not yet been absorbed; of these, most have already moved close to the upper barrier. The overall probability to absorb at the upper barrier (0.790) is equal to the total area under g_+; similarly, the area (0.210) under g_- corresponds to the overall probability to absorb at the lower barrier. The conditional mean first-passage time is 223 for the upper and 50 for the lower barrier

As we will see, with two barriers, the basic solutions for $f(x, t|a, b)$ generally take the form of infinite series. Therefore, the formal mathematical apparatus is more elaborate than in the case of a single barrier, and we must borrow some pertinent formal results.

One standard approach is to assume that f can be *separated*, that is, be written as a product $f(x, t|a, b) = v(x) \cdot w(t)$, say. Inserting this separation approach into the forward Equation (4.18) then gives

$$v(x)\, w'(t) = \left[\frac{1}{2}\sigma^2 v''(x) - \mu v'(x)\right] w(t) \qquad \text{or}$$

$$\frac{w'(t)}{w(t)} = \frac{\frac{1}{2}\sigma^2 v''(x) - \mu v'(x)}{v(x)} \tag{4.52}$$

Equation (4.52) must hold for all t and x, and its left-hand side is independent of x, whereas its right-hand side is independent of t. Therefore, both sides of the equation are equal to some constant, say, $-\lambda$. This is perhaps easiest seen if one thinks of taking the derivative of Eq. (4.52) with respect to x and to t which would in both cases produce zero. Thus, w and v must separately satisfy a linear ordinary differential equation of the first (as for w) and of the second (as for v) order

$$\lambda\, w(t) + w'(t) = 0 \tag{4.53}$$

$$\lambda v(x) - \mu v'(x) + \frac{1}{2}\sigma^2 v''(x) = 0 \tag{4.54}$$

the solutions of which are standard (e.g., Stewart 2012, ch.s 9 and 17). It is then not difficult to confirm that for integer values of n, any function of the general form

$$f_n(x, t) = \exp\left(\frac{\mu x}{\sigma^2} - \lambda_n t\right) \sin\left[\frac{n\pi}{a+b}(x+b)\right] \tag{4.55}$$

will satisfy the boundary conditions $f(-b, t) = f(a, t) = 0$ because the term $\sin\left[\frac{n\pi}{a+b}(x+b)\right] = 0$ for $x = -b$ and for $x = a$. Furthermore, it is straightforward to check from Eq. (4.18) that the functions $f_n(x, t)$ will satisfy the forward equation provided that

$$\lambda_n = \frac{1}{2}\left[\left(\frac{\mu}{\sigma}\right)^2 + \left(\frac{n\pi\sigma}{a+b}\right)^2\right] \tag{4.56}$$

This means that we can superimpose weighted solutions f_n for $n = 1, 2, \ldots$ so as to also satisfy the initial condition for f as $t \to 0$. This is a standard exercise in the theory of Fourier series (e.g., Wylie and Barrett 1995, ch. 8); the customary approach exploits the orthogonality properties of the sin function and shows that on choosing the coefficients c_n as

$$c_n = \frac{2}{a+b} \sin\left(\frac{n\pi b}{a+b}\right) \tag{4.57}$$

the transition density function may be represented as

$$f(x, t | a, b) = \sum_{n=1}^{\infty} c_n \cdot f_n(x, t) \tag{4.58}$$

The series representation of f in Eq. (4.58) converges for all $t > 0$. However, the rate of convergence can be slow for small values of t, especially when σ is small and a and b are large. For practical work, it is therefore useful to have an alternative representation of f that converges faster for small t.

The obtain an alternative representation of the transition density f, it is helpful to reconsider the manner in which we obtained in Sect. 4.2.1 a transition density that conformed to the corresponding boundary condition in the single-barrier case. We first noted that normal densities with variance $\sigma^2 t$ generally obey the forward equation (cf., Eq. (3.8)) and also conform to the initial condition as $t \to 0$. We then choose a suitable linear combination (i.e., Eq. (4.20)) of two such normal densities to satisfy the boundary condition Eq. (4.19) as well. In a sense, this approach is complementary to the separation approach leading to the Fourier series Eq. (4.58). Specifically, the separation approach is based on individual solutions f_n as in Eq. (4.55) which all satisfy the boundary conditions and which are then aggregated so as to satisfy the initial condition as well. In contrast, the approach involving normal densities is based on individual solutions which all satisfy the initial condition at $t = 0$ and which are then aggregated so as to satisfy the boundary conditions as well.

More specifically, a normal density with variance $\sigma^2 t$ centered on $x = 0$ satisfies the initial condition but not the boundary condition at a and $-b$. Therefore, much as we did in Sect. 4.2.1, we subtract another normal density centered on $x = 2a$ which for reasons of symmetry cancels the contribution of the first density at $x = a$. Similarly, we subtract a normal density centered on $x = -2b$ which cancels the contribution of the first density at $x = -b$. The first of these additions, however, requires a further addition of a normal component centered on $x = -2(a + b)$ to satisfy the condition at $x = -b$; similarly, the second addition requires the addition of a normal component centered on $x = 2(a + b)$, and so forth. Continuing this approach of successive cancellations eventually leads to the alternative representation of the transition density

$$f(x, t|a, b) = \exp\left(\frac{\mu x}{\sigma^2} - \frac{\mu^2 t}{2\sigma^2}\right) \cdot$$

$$\sum_{n=-\infty}^{\infty} \left[n(x|2n(a+b), \sigma^2 t) - n(x|2a - 2n(a+b), \sigma^2 t) \right] \tag{4.59}$$

where $n(x|u, v^2)$ is the normal density with mean u and variance v^2. Note that when t is small, essentially only the first few summands for which the index $|n|$ of the sum is small will contribute to x–values in the interval $[-b, a]$ in which we are interested. This means that Eq. (4.59) will typically converge soon when t is small. Together with Eq. (4.58), we then have two (mathematically equivalent) representations of $f(x, t|a, b)$ which converge fairly quickly in their respective domains.

Similar to our approach in Sect. 4.2.1, we define as $G(t|a, b)$ the probability that $\mathbf{T}_{ab} > t$. Note that $G(t|a, b) = G_+(t|a, b) + G_-(t|a, b)$ because the events to absorb at $x = -b$ or at $x = a$ are mutually exclusive, so that their probabilities add. This also means that the corresponding first-passage time density $g(t|a, b) = g_+(t|a, b) + g_-(t|a, b)$.

As illustrated in Fig. 4.8, the basic relation between f and G, corresponding to Eq. (4.21) in the one-barrier scenario, then is

$$1 - G(t|a, b) = \int_{-b}^{a} f(x, t|a, b)\, dx \tag{4.60}$$

We next differentiate this equation with respect to t and then use the fact that f satisfies the forward equation (4.18). Following similar steps as in the derivation of Eq. (4.23), we get

$$g(t|a, b) = -\frac{1}{2}\sigma^2 \frac{\partial}{\partial x} f(x, t|a, b)\Big|_{x=-b}^{x=a} + \mu\, f(x, t|a, b)\Big|_{x=-b}^{x=a}$$

The evaluation of the second term $f(x, t|a, b)$ at $x = -b$ and at $x = a$ equals zero because of the boundary condition Eq. (4.51) for the absorbing barriers. This leaves us with the result

$$g(t|a, b) = -\frac{1}{2}\sigma^2 \frac{\partial}{\partial x} f(x, t|a, b)\Big|_{x=a} + \frac{1}{2}\sigma^2 \frac{\partial}{\partial x} f(x, t|a, b)\Big|_{x=-b} \tag{4.61}$$

Considering the first summand, we recall from Eq. (4.13) that the flux of probability across a boundary at x is generally given as

$$J(x, t) = -\frac{1}{2}\sigma^2 \frac{\partial}{\partial x} f(x, t|a, b) + \mu\, f(x, t|a, b)$$

Focusing, specifically, on $x = a$, the boundary condition is $f(a, t|a, b) = 0$, and so we get for the flux across $x = a$, that is, for the contribution to g specifically from absorptions at the upper barrier,

$$g_+(t|a, b) = J(a, t) = -\frac{1}{2}\sigma^2 \frac{\partial}{\partial x} f(x, t|a, b)\Big|_{x=a} \tag{4.62}$$

Equation (4.62) corresponds precisely to the first summand on the right-hand side of Eq. (4.61) and represents the first-passage time density g_+ for absorptions at the upper barrier a.

At the lower barrier, to obtain g_-, we need to consider the flux of probability in the right-to-left direction across $x = -b$, which inverts the sign of our standard (left-to-right) flux expression, Eq. (4.13). We thus get for the first-passage time density at the lower barrier

$$g_-(x, t|a, b) = -J(-b, t) = \frac{1}{2}\sigma^2 \frac{\partial}{\partial x} f(x, t|a, b)\Big|_{x=-b} \tag{4.63}$$

which in turn corresponds to the second summand on the right-hand side of Eq. (4.61), representing the first-passage time density g_- for absorptions at the lower barrier $-b$.

In summary, $g(t|a, b)$ in Eq. (4.61) gives the overall density to absorb at time t. The first summand on the right-hand side of Eq. (4.61) represents the density $g_+(t|a, b)$ for the joint event to absorb at t and at the upper barrier a; the second summand is the corresponding density $g_-(t|a, b)$ for the joint event to absorb at t and at the lower barrier $-b$.

It remains to carry out the differentiation of f indicated in Eqs. (4.62) and (4.63). Corresponding to the representation of f in Eq. (4.58), we get for $g_+(t|a, b)$ the Fourier series solution

$$g_+(t|a, b) = \pi \left(\frac{\sigma}{a+b}\right)^2 \exp\left(\frac{a\mu}{\sigma^2}\right) \sum_{n=1}^{\infty} n \sin\left(\frac{n\pi a}{a+b}\right) \exp(-\lambda_n t)$$

$$\text{where} \quad \lambda_n = \frac{1}{2}\left[\left(\frac{\mu}{\sigma}\right)^2 + \left(\frac{n\pi\sigma}{a+b}\right)^2\right] \tag{4.64}$$

As discussed above, this series converges for all $t > 0$, but the rate of convergence is slow for small values of t, especially when σ is small and a and b are large.

For practical work, it is therefore useful to have a second representation of g_+ which converges faster for small t. To this end, we carry out the differentiation indicated in Eq. (4.62) based on the alternative representation of f in Eq. (4.59), which leads to the alternative representation

$$g_+(t|a, b) = \frac{\sigma}{2\sqrt{2\pi t}} \sum_{n=-\infty}^{\infty} a_n(t) \exp[b_n(t)] - c_n(t) \exp[d_n(t)] \qquad (4.65)$$

$$a_n(t) = \frac{a - 2n(a + b) - \mu t}{\sigma^2 t}$$

$$b_n(t) = \frac{2\mu n(a + b)}{\sigma^2} - \frac{(a - 2n(a + b) - \mu t)^2}{2\sigma^2 t}$$

$$c_n(t) = \frac{-a + 2n(a + b) - \mu t}{\sigma^2 t}$$

$$d_n(t) = \frac{2\mu[a - n(a + b)]}{\sigma^2} - \frac{(-a + 2n(a + b) - \mu t)^2}{2\sigma^2 t}$$

Writing more explicitly $g_+(t|a, b) = g_+(t|\mu, \sigma^2, a, b)$, the first-passage time density g_- for the absorption at the lower barrier $-b$ is obtained by the evident symmetry relation

$$g_-(t|\mu, \sigma^2, a, b) = g_+(t| - \mu, \sigma^2, b, a) \qquad (4.66)$$

For example, the distribution of the time to reach the *upper* barrier when $a = 10, -b = -5$, and $\mu = 1$ is necessarily the same as the time to reach the *lower* barrier when $a = 5, -b = -10$, and $\mu = -1$.

Figure 4.9 shows the densities g_+ and g_- for the values $\mu = 1, \sigma = 8, a = 250$, and $-b = -50$. As explained in Fig. 4.8, for these parameters, a proportion of about 0.79 of all paths absorb at the upper barrier. The positive drift and the relative distance of the barriers to the starting point at 0 mean that the lower barrier is nearly exclusively reached during the early phases of the diffusion process. At later stages, the positive drift becomes dominant, and returns to the region close to the lower barrier are increasingly improbable. In effect, for the scenario shown in Fig. 4.8, absorptions at $-b$ take place either early on or never. For example, the conditional mean first-passage time for absorptions the lower barrier is 50, as compared to 223 for absorptions the upper barrier.

4.4.4 Moment-Generating Functions for Two Barriers

In Sect. 4.2.3, we saw that for a Wiener process $X(t)$ starting at $X(0) = 0$, the mgf of the first-passage time to $a > 0$ is

$$m^+(s|a) = \mathsf{E}[\exp(-sT_a)] = \exp\left[\frac{a}{\sigma^2}\left(\mu - \sqrt{2s\sigma^2 + \mu^2}\right)\right] \qquad (4.67)$$

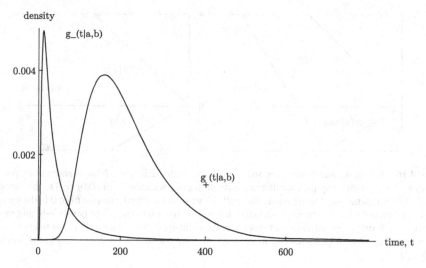

Fig. 4.9 The first-passage time densities (ordinate) $g_-(t|a, b)$ (left) and $g_+(t|a, b)$ (right) for $\mu = 1, \sigma = 8, a = 250$, and $b = 50$; for their genesis, see Fig. 4.8. The areas under these densities represent the overall probabilities of about 0.79 and 0.21 to absorb at the upper or lower barrier, respectively

where we have added to m a superscript to indicate that the barrier is placed *above* the starting point. We derived this result from the corresponding pgf for the simple random walk and assumed that $\mu > 0$. The derivation remains in fact valid when $\mu < 0$ (and still $a > 0$), but we must take care to interpret the root correctly, because for a negative number μ, we have $\sqrt{\mu^2} = -\mu$. Specifically, for $\mu < 0$, we get for the probability of ever reaching the barrier $m^+(s = 0|a) = \exp\left(\frac{2a\mu}{\sigma^2}\right) < 1$, correctly indicating that when the drift is negative, a fraction of $1 - m^+(s = 0|a)$ of all paths will never reach $a > 0$.

We next consider how these results for the mgf—which in this case we write as m^-—are modified when the barrier is *below* the starting point $x = 0$. For symmetry reasons, for a drift μ, the distribution of first-passage times to the barrier $x = -b < 0$, and thus the associated mgf, must be the same as the distribution of first-passage times to $x = +b > 0$ for a drift of $-\mu$, where the latter mgf m^+ is given by Eq. (4.67). Replacing μ with $-\mu$ in Eq. (4.67), we conclude that for a barrier at $-b < 0$, the mgf takes the form

$$m^-(s|b) = \mathrm{E}[\exp(-s\mathbf{T}_{-b})] = \exp\left[\frac{b}{\sigma^2}\left(-\mu - \sqrt{2s\sigma^2 + \mu^2}\right)\right] \quad (4.68)$$

Note that as expected $m^-(s = 0|b) = 1$ when $\mu < 0$, but $m^-(s = 0|b) = \exp\left(-\frac{2b\mu}{\sigma^2}\right) < 1$ when $\mu > 0$. The important point here is that the form of the mgfs m^+ and m^- differs for barriers placed above and below the starting point $x = 0$.

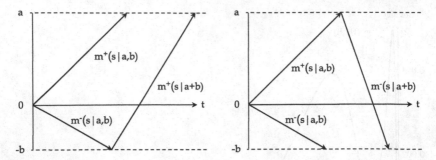

Fig. 4.10 Abscissa, time t; ordinates, spatial position, with barriers at $-b$ and a and starting point at $x_0 = 0$. Left panel: any path leading in the single-barrier scenario from $X(0) = 0$ to the barrier $a > 0$ either reaches this barrier before the level $-b$ was ever reached (the line from 0 to the upper barrier a) or first reaches the level $-b$ before a (the line from 0 to the lower barrier $-b$) and then moves $a + b$ units upward to reach the level a (the right-most line). The right panel refers to the corresponding case of paths leading in the single-barrier scenario from $X(0) = 0$ to the barrier $-b < 0$

We dwell on these somewhat subtle points because the mgfs m^+, m^- for the single-barrier scenario can be used to obtain, in an elementary manner, the mgfs of the conditional first-passage time densities g_+ and g_- in the two-barrier scenario. In the following, we denote the mgfs referring to the two-barrier scenario as $m^+(s|a, b)$ (for absorptions at the upper barrier $a > 0$) and $m^-(s|a, b)$ (for absorptions at the lower barrier $-b < 0$); note that mgfs for the two-barrier scenario are distinguished by carrying two arguments after the | line.

The reasoning to obtain $m^+(s|a, b)$ and $m^-(s|a, b)$ corresponds essentially to the argument that we have used before in Sects. 2.3.2 and 2.3.3 for simple random walks (see Figs. 2.6 and 2.7) and is illustrated in Fig. 4.10, replacing for more clarity noisy sample paths by straight lines.

Any path leading in the single-barrier scenario from $X(0) = 0$ to the barrier $a > 0$ belongs to one of two mutually exclusive and exhaustive classes, illustrated in the left part of Figure 4.10. Either (i) the barrier a is reached before the level $-b$ was ever reached before, as shown by the line from 0 to the upper barrier a, or (ii) the level $-b$ was reached before a (the line from 0 to the lower barrier $-b$), followed by an upward passage of $a + b$ units to reach the level a (the right-most line). The first passages illustrated by the two lines starting at 0 refer to the two-barrier scenario, whereas the right-most line in the left panel refers to a single-barrier scenario. The case (i) refers to the first-passage time to a in the two-barrier scenario (with mgf $m^+(s|a, b)$) and the case (ii) to a first-passage to $-b$ (with mgf $m^-(s|a, b)$) in the two-barrier scenario, followed by a first-passage from $-b$ to a (with mgf $m^+(s|a + b)$) in the single-barrier scenario. Because the mgf of the sum of two random variables (i.e., the first-passage from 0 to $-b$, plus the first-passage from there to a) equals the product of their individual mgfs, we get Eq. (4.69). The corresponding Eq. (4.70) is derived by the same reasoning.

$$m^+(s|a) = m^+(s|a, b) + m^-(s|a, b) \cdot m^+(s|a+b) \qquad (4.69)$$

$$m^-(s|b) = m^-(s|a, b) + m^+(s|a, b) \cdot m^-(s|a+b) \qquad (4.70)$$

These are two linear equations in the two unknowns $m^+(s|a, b)$ and $m^-(s|a, b)$, which can be solved in terms of the known mgfs referring to the two single-barrier scenarios, as given by Eqs. (4.67) and (4.68). We get

$$m^+(s|a, b) = \frac{m^+(s|a) - m^-(s|b) \cdot m^+(s|a+b)}{1 - m^+(s|a+b) \cdot m^-(s|a+b)} \qquad (4.71)$$

$$m^-(s|a, b) = \frac{m^-(s|b) - m^+(s|a) \cdot m^-(s|a+b)}{1 - m^+(s|a+b) \cdot m^-(s|a+b)} \qquad (4.72)$$

For explicit results, see, for example, Darling and Siegert (1953). The results for $m^+(s|a, b)$ and $m^+(s|a, b)$ may in turn be used to extract absorption probabilities and conditional moments of the first-passage times.

For the case $a = b$, the results are easily derived and especially instructive. They show that when $a = b$, the mgfs, when conditioned on absorbing at their respective barrier, are identical,

$$\frac{m^+(s|a, a)}{m^+(0|a, a)} = \frac{m^-(s|a, a)}{m^-(0|a, a)}$$

This means that the conditional first-passage time densities g_+/p_a and g_-/p_{-a} are identical in this special case. In fact, for $a = b$, we obtain from Eqs. (4.71) and (4.72) the common conditional mgf of these first-passage times explicitly as

$$\frac{m^+(s|a, a)}{m^+(0|a, a)} = \frac{m^-(s|a, a)}{m^-(0|a, a)} = \frac{\cosh\left(\frac{a\mu}{\sigma^2}\right)}{\cosh\left(\frac{a}{\sigma^2}\sqrt{\mu^2 + 2s\sigma^2}\right)} \qquad (4.73)$$

In view of Eq. (4.44) for the absorption probability $\psi(\mu, \sigma^2|a, a)$, we may for equally distant barriers conclude that when the drift μ is positive (negative), then the process absorbs more often at the upper (lower) barrier, but the time to absorption has the same distribution for either barrier.

4.5 Two Reflecting Barriers

In the case of two reflecting barriers, there is by definition no escape from the interval between the boundaries at $-b$ and a. The basic quantity of interest in this case is the transition density $f(x, t)$ for the process to be at x at time t; because of the spatial homogeneity of the Wiener process, we may without loss of generality assume that the start is at $X(0) = 0$. When both barriers are reflecting, no probability can flow off across the boundaries, and so f must integrate to 1 at all times t. As before, f is narrowly concentrated at 0 as $t \to 0$, and it satisfies the forward Equation (4.18) in the variables x and t. However, it must in addition satisfy the zero-flux condition at both reflecting boundaries,

$$J(a, t) = J(-b, t) = 0 \qquad \text{for } t > 0 \tag{4.74}$$

where the flux $J(x, t)$ is defined in Eq. (4.13). The techniques to solve the forward equation under these initial and boundary conditions closely parallel those for two absorbing barriers. They will not be reproduced here; explicit solutions can be found, for example, in Sweet and Hardin (1970); see also Schwarz and Stein (1998).

Given that f integrates at all times to 1, it is natural to expect that as t increases, it converges to a limiting, stationary form that is independent of t and of x_0. It is thus of interest to determine this stationary density which we denote as $f^*(x)$. By the notion of stationarity, the density f will not change any more with t, which means that f^* is a solution of Eq. (4.18) for $\frac{\partial f}{\partial t} = 0$. Therefore, we set to zero the forward equation

$$\frac{\partial f}{\partial t} = \frac{1}{2}\sigma^2 \frac{\partial^2 f}{\partial x^2} - \mu \frac{\partial f}{\partial x} = 0$$

and thus get a simple first-order equation for $\frac{\partial f^*}{\partial x}$ which must be solved under the boundary conditions given in Eq. (4.74).

This approach gives the stationary solution

$$f^*(x) = \frac{\frac{2\mu}{\sigma^2} \exp\left(\frac{2\mu x}{\sigma^2}\right)}{\exp\left(\frac{2\mu a}{\sigma^2}\right) - \exp\left(-\frac{2\mu b}{\sigma^2}\right)} \tag{4.75}$$

which is an exponential density with rate $2\mu/\sigma^2$, censored to the interval $[-b, a]$. The form of the stationary density f^* in Eq. (4.75) has several features much as we would expect. For example, if $\mu > 0$, then f^* increases toward the right (upper) barrier a, whereas for $\mu < 0$, it tends toward the left (lower) barrier at $-b$. The concentration toward the respective boundary will be stronger the smaller the σ^2 is. For $\mu \to 0$, the stationary density tends to the uniform distribution $f^*(x) = 1/(a+b)$ over the interval $[-b, a]$.

4.6 The Mixed Case: One Absorbing and One Reflecting Barrier

The final combination of the status of the upper and lower barrier confining a Wiener process concerns the case of one reflecting barrier, at $-b$ say, and one absorbing barrier at a. The transition density $f(x, t)$ must then satisfy the zero-flux condition at $x = -b$ and the zero-density condition at $x = a$, that is,

$$J(-b, t) = 0 \quad \text{and} \quad f(a, t) = 0 \quad \text{for } t > 0 \quad (4.76)$$

where the flux $J(x, t)$ is defined in Eq. (4.13).

It is clear that there is then only a single first-passage time density, $g_+(t|a, b)$, which is regular (i.e., it integrates to 1 across t) because probability flows off only across the barrier at $x = a$. As in Eq. (4.62), the first-passage time density g_+ is related to the transition density f via the flux across $x = a$,

$$g_+(t|a, b) = -\frac{1}{2}\sigma^2 f(x, t)\Big|_{x=a} \quad (4.77)$$

The techniques to solve the forward Equation (4.18) under the boundary conditions described by Eq. (4.76) resemble those for two absorbing barriers applied in Sect. 4.4.3, but present some additional analytical complications. They are described in detail in Schwarz (1992) to which we refer for explicit complete solutions and further discussion. In Sect. 6.4, we will consider how to find the mean first-passage time to the absorbing barrier at a for the Wiener and also for more complex processes.

4.7 The Backward Process

So far, we have analyzed the evolution of the Wiener process prospectively, that is, looking forward in time. Specifically, the transition density f is initially assumed to be narrowly concentrated around the starting point x_0, and the forward Equation (4.18) then describes the evolution of the diffusion process in time and space, under boundary conditions appropriate to the problem at hand. In some situations, it is, however, of interest to look, retrospectively, back in time and to study the course of events that has led up to the absorption at a given barrier. To this end, we define the *backward process* which, in the specific case considered here, is a simple transformation of an underlying Wiener process $\{X(t), t \geq 0\}$. We assume that $X(t)$ has positive drift $\mu > 0$ and starts at $X(0) = 0$ in the presence of a single absorbing barrier at $a > 0$.

The construction of a backward process is motivated by applications which observe an empirical time series up to a specific terminating event, such as death or some other well-defined binary response. Time series of this character may sometimes be interpreted as resulting from an underlying diffusion process leading up to the crossing of some critical level, a (for details and applications, see Sect. 7.2). One technique designed to study the dynamics of the approach toward the terminating event is known as "response locking" the time series to the level crossing. The basic idea is to temporally re-align the original observed time series by taking the moment $\mathbf{T}_a$ at which the threshold a is first reached as time zero. It is then possible to look at the time series "backward" from this moment on. Essentially, we are asking then: what is the probability that t time units before it absorbed at a the process was at some specific position y below the threshold a?

To study the properties of this construction, we formally define the backward process as $Y(t) \equiv X(\mathbf{T}_a - t)$. Loosely speaking, $Y(\cdot)$ is essentially just $X(\cdot)$, but as seen "backward", from the moment $\mathbf{T}_a$ of the first-passage through a. Some properties of $Y(t)$ immediately follow from this definition. For example, it must be the case that $Y(0) = a$; also, necessarily $Y(t) < a$ for $t > 0$.

It is important to note that for a given t, the random variable $Y(t)$ is defined only in the case of $\mathbf{T}_a \geq t$: we cannot look backward for a time that is longer than it took the original process to reach a for the first time. This implies that for any fixed t, the distribution of $Y(t)$ has a defect (it does not integrate to 1), and this defect is, by the construction of the process $Y(t)$, just equal to $P(\mathbf{T}_a < t) = G(t|a)$, where the density g corresponding to G is given in Eq. (4.22). Therefore, in any computation related to $Y(t)$ (e.g., its density or its expectation), we can account for this defect by conditioning on that subsample of paths of the original process $X(\cdot)$ which took at least t time units to first reach the barrier at a.

We next obtain a simple relation to find the density, say $k(y, t)$, of $Y(t)$, where $t > 0$ is an arbitrary but fixed index of the time as measured looking backward from the moment of absorption at a and $y < a$. Put simple, $k(y, t)$ is the density that t time units before it absorbed at a the process $X(\cdot)$ was at position $y < a$. By the definition of $Y(t)$, we have, indicating densities in the presence of an absorbing barrier at a by the index a,

$$k(y, t) = P_a[Y(t) = y] = P_a[X(\mathbf{T}_a - t) = y] \qquad (4.78)$$

In order for the event $Y(t) = y$ to occur, only the cases of $\mathbf{T}_a \geq t$ can contribute; conditioning on the value, say v, of the first-passage time $\mathbf{T}_a$, we get

$$k(y, t) = \int_t^\infty P_a[X(v - t) = y | \mathbf{T}_a = v] \cdot P_a[\mathbf{T}_a = v] \, dv \qquad (4.79)$$

The expression $P_a[X(v - t) = y | \mathbf{T}_a = v]$ refers to the event that the position of the original process $X(\cdot)$ at time $v - t$ was y, given that t time units later (i.e., at time v), the process absorbed at a. We observe that the integrand $P_a[X(v - t) = y | \mathbf{T}_a = v] \cdot P_a[\mathbf{T}_a = v]$ appearing in Eq. (4.79) is of the general form $P(E_1|E_2) \cdot P(E_2)$ where E_1 and E_2 represent two events with $P(E_2) > 0$.

As for the event denoted as E_2, we know that for $v > 0$, the first-passage time T_a has the density $g(v|a)$ given by Eq. (4.22). According to elementary standard relations among conditional probabilities (i.e., Bayes' theorem), an equivalent way of writing the integrand in Eq. (4.79) is $P(E_2|E_1) \cdot P(E_1)$, which gives

$$k(y, t) = \int_t^\infty P_a[T_a = v | X(v - t) = y] \cdot P_a[X(v - t) = y] \, dv \qquad (4.80)$$

We next consider in turn the functions contributing to the product in the integrand of Eq. (4.79).

First, the expression $P_a[T_a = v | X(v - t) = y]$ in Eq. (4.80) refers to the event that the original Wiener process $X(\cdot)$ reaches the level a for the first time at time $v > t$ given that t time units before (i.e., at time $v - t$), it was at position $y < a$. We know that the Wiener process is homogeneous in time and space, as is evident from the transition density Eq. (4.17). This means that the expression $P_a[T_a = v | X(v - t) = y]$ depends only on the temporal separation of the two events $\{T_a = v\}$ and $\{X(v - t) = y\}$, that is, on $v - (v - t) = t$, and on the spatial distance to the barrier, $a - y$, but not on the variable v. Thus, for any values of y and t, and regardless of v, $P_a[T_a = v | X(v - t) = y]$ refers to an event that is equivalent to starting from $x = 0$ and reaching a barrier placed at $a - y$ first at time t. This means that the first factor $P_a[T_a = v | X(v - t) = y]$ is equal to the first-passage time density $g(t | a - y)$, with g given by Eq. (4.22).

The second factor in the integrand of Eq. (4.80) is the regular transition density $f(y, v - t | a)$ of the Wiener process in the presence of an absorbing barrier at a, namely, the density f as given by Eq. (4.20) for the original process $X(\cdot)$ to be at position y at time $v - t$ when an absorbing barrier is placed at a. Inserting these facts, we obtain

$$k(y, t) = \int_t^\infty g(t | a - y) \cdot f(y, v - t | a) \, dv \qquad (4.81)$$

Moving factors independent of the integration variable v out of the integral, and changing the integration variable to $w = v - t$, $dv = dw$, we finally obtain the basic relation

$$k(y, t) = g(t | a - y) \cdot \int_0^\infty f(y, w | a) \, dw \qquad (4.82)$$

with g given by Eq. (4.22) and f by Eq. (4.20).

In hindsight at least, this result seems plausible. For $Y(t)$ to be equal to some value $y < a$, it must be the case that, firstly, the original process $X(\cdot)$ was at some arbitrary time $w > 0$ at position $X(w) = y$ when an absorbing barrier is placed at

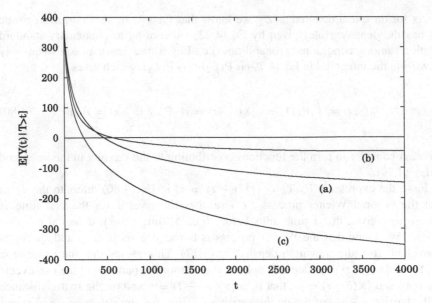

Fig. 4.11 Conditional means $E[Y(t)|T_a \geq t]$ (ordinate) of the backward process $Y(t)$ as a function of t (abscissa) for $a = 400$ and three parameter combinations $< \mu, \sigma >:$ $< 1, 15 >$ **(a)**, $< 2, 15 >$ **(b)**, and $< 1, 20 >$ **(c)**

a and that, secondly, exactly t time units later $X(\cdot)$ then absorbed at a. Integrating across all possible values of w, we get $k(y, t)$.

As explained, the unconditional density k has a defect, equal to $G(t|a)$. If we condition on the event $T_a \geq t$, then we get the regular conditional density

$$k^*(y, t) = \frac{k(y, t)}{1 - G(t|a)} \tag{4.83}$$

For explicit analytical results related to the density k^* and several further results describing the backward process $Y(t)$, see Schwarz and Miller (2010).

Figure 4.11 shows the conditional expectation $E[Y(t)|T_a \geq t]$ of the backward process for an absorbing barrier placed at $a = 400$ under three different parameter combinations. In all three cases, two features stand out: (i) the initial decline of $E[Y(t)|T_a \geq t]$ is quite steep, and (ii) its asymptotic level is negative.

Considering that the original Wiener process started from $X(0) = 0$ and is characterized by a positive drift rate, the feature (ii) seems quite remarkable. This phenomenon is not due, as one might suspect, to conditioning on rather extreme regions of the distribution of T_a. For example, for the case (a) of $a = 400$, $\mu = 1$, and $\sigma = 15$ depicted in Fig. 4.11, the conditional expectation of $Y(t)$ turns negative at $t = 468$, at a time when a proportion of $1 - G(t|a) = 0.286$ of all sample paths of $X(\cdot)$ is not yet absorbed at a and thus contributes to the conditional expectation. In fact, for many other parameter combinations, $E[Y(t)|T_a \geq t]$ turns negative much earlier, relative to the distribution of $\mathbf{T}_a$. Thus, the negative conditional expectation of $Y(t)$ is not a phenomenon that occurs only for extreme regions of the process where only few, untypical sample paths contribute to form the expectation, but is a feature of rather central, representative portions of the distribution of $\mathbf{T}_a$.

Of similar interest is the feature (i), the steep initial decline of $E[Y(t)|\mathbf{T}_a \geq t]$ for small values of t, when $G(t|a)$ is still very close to zero so that essentially all sample paths of $X(\cdot)$ contribute to the conditional expectation. For example, for the case (a) of $a = 400$, $\mu = 1$, and $\sigma = 15$ in Fig. 4.11, we have that $G(t|a) = 2.2 \cdot 10^{-16}$ for $t = 10$, meaning that with these parameters, essentially all first passages to a take more than 10 time units. Looking back 10 time units from the moment $\mathbf{T}_a$ of absorption at $a = 400$, the conditional expectation is found to be equal to $E[Y(10)|\mathbf{T}_a \geq 10] = 323.7$. This value means that on average during the last 10 time units before absorption at $a = 400$ took place, a remaining distance of $400 - 323.7 = 76.3$ is crossed, as compared with the "regular" displacement of only $\mu \cdot t = 10$ during a time interval of this length.

Both of these features, although quite counter-intuitive at first, faithfully reflect elementary properties of the underlying Wiener process. Specifically, the fact that the conditional expectation $E[Y(t)|\mathbf{T}_a \geq t]$ falls below the starting value as t increases is not evidence for some negative drift component but corresponds precisely to what is expected for an underlying Wiener process. Loosely speaking, by conditioning on $\mathbf{T}_a \geq t$, for large t, we essentially select for those sample paths which happened to take a particularly long time to reach a. Almost by definition, for those paths, it is common to show large excursions to regions well below their starting points—or else they would have been absorbed by that time.

Similarly, the steep initial decrease of $E[Y(t)|\mathbf{T}_a \geq t]$ in t does per se not represent evidence of some emergent "final pull" or other attracting, accelerating force that suddenly starts to drive $X(\cdot)$ toward the terminating event. Rather, by looking backward t time units from the moment of the first passage to a, when t is small, we select for those specific subsets of all sample paths which happened to make particularly large positive excursions and thereby passed a. Thus, both features (i) and (ii) shown in Fig. 4.11 are in perfect agreement with what we should expect when the underlying mechanism generating the observed time series conforms to an ordinary Wiener process.

4.8 Exercises

1. Note and explain the close analogy between the pair of forward and backward equations 2.3 and 2.4 for the simple random walk and the corresponding pair of Eqs. 4.12 and 4.16. Use the limit relations Eq. (4.9) to derive the latter pair of equations directly from the former pair. In Sect. 2.2.2, we observed that for $p = \frac{1}{2}$, the structure of the forward and backward equation for the simple random walk is formally identical but that these equations refer to different spatial variables. How does this translate to the Wiener process?

2. Show that if $f(x, t)$ is the transition density of a diffusion process starting at x_0, satisfying the forward equation

$$\frac{\partial f}{\partial t} = \frac{1}{2}\sigma^2 \frac{\partial^2 f}{\partial x^2} - \mu \frac{\partial f}{\partial x}$$

then the function

$$g(x, t) = f(x, t) \cdot \exp\left[-\frac{2\mu(x - x_0) - \mu^2 t}{2\sigma^2}\right]$$

satisfies the simpler equation

$$\frac{\partial g}{\partial t} = \frac{1}{2}\sigma^2 \frac{\partial^2 g}{\partial x^2}$$

solutions of which are well-known from classical heat conduction theory.

3. It is readily seen that for the function g as defined in Exercise 2, the boundary condition $f(a, t) = 0$ for an absorbing barrier at $x = a$ translates into $g(a, t) = 0$. Show that for a *reflecting* barrier, the boundary condition (4.38) at $x = a$ translates into

$$\left.\frac{\partial g}{\partial x}\right|_{x=a} = \frac{\mu}{\sigma^2} g(a, t)$$

4. Use Eq. (4.34) to show that the mean and variance of the density $g(t|a, x_0)$ given in Eq. (4.24) are $E[T_a] = (a - x_0)/\mu$ and $Var[T_a] = a\sigma^2/\mu^3$, respectively. To this end, use the cumulant generating function which is the natural logarithm of the mgf; its first and second derivatives at $s = 0$ give directly the (negative of the) mean and the variance. Show that $E[T_a]$ corresponds (with $x_0 = 0$) to the limit of $b \to -\infty$ in Eq. (4.46).

5. Use the absorption probability Eq. (4.44) and the form of the first-passage time density in Eq. (4.66) to explain that for $a = b$, the first-passage time has the same density conditional on absorbing at the upper or lower barrier.

6. Conclude from Eqs. (4.48) and (4.49) that for $a = b$, the conditional mean first-passage times to either barrier are identical and may be written as

$$E[T] = \frac{a}{\mu} \cdot \tanh\left(\frac{a\mu}{\sigma^2}\right)$$

Confirm this result starting from Eq. (4.73); use the cumulant generating function defined in Exercise 4. Interpret the factor $\tanh\left(\frac{a\mu}{\sigma^2}\right)$ by comparing to the corresponding result for the mean first-passage time to a in the single-barrier scenario (Exercise 4).

7. Use Eq. (4.73) to show that for equally distant barriers $a = b$, the variance of the first-passage time to either barrier is given by

$$\text{Var}[\mathbf{T}] = \frac{a\sigma^2}{\mu^3} \cdot \left(\tanh(k) - \frac{k}{\cosh^2(k)} \right) \quad , \quad \text{where} \quad k = \frac{a\mu}{\sigma^2}$$

As in the previous Exercise 6, interpret the $(\ldots)$ expression to the right of $a\sigma^2/\mu^3$ by comparing to the corresponding result of Exercise 4 for the variance of the first-passage time to a in the single-barrier scenario. Investigate and interpret the behavior of this expression as a function of $k = a\mu/\sigma^2$.

8. Starting from the basic relation Eq. (4.21), show by direct integration of f, as given by Eq. (4.20), that

$$P(\mathbf{T}_a > t) = 1 - G(t|a) = \Phi\left(\frac{a - \mu t}{\sigma \sqrt{t}} \right) - \exp\left(\frac{2\mu a}{\sigma^2} \right) \Phi\left(-\frac{\mu t + a}{\sigma \sqrt{t}} \right)$$

where $t > 0$ and Φ is the standard normal distribution function. Verify that the derivative of $G(t|a)$ with respect to t corresponds to the first-passage time density $g(t|a)$ as given in Eq. (4.22).

9. The density $g(t|a)$ in Eq. (4.22) is often called the *inverse Gaussian* distribution. The reason for this name is a relation between the cumulant generating function (see Exercise 4) of the density for the unrestricted motion of a Wiener process and that of the first-passage time associated with it.

   Use Eq. (3.12) to find the cumulant generating function of the (normal) density of $X(t)$ in a Wiener process with drift μ and variance parameter σ^2. From the basic properties of the Wiener process, such as Eqs. (4.5) and (4.6), this function must be proportional to t; thus, write it in the form of $t \cdot u(s)$. Similarly, use Eq. (4.34) to find the cumulant generating function of the first-passage time density to the level a. By the additivity of first-passage times, this function must be proportional to a; thus, write it in the form of $a \cdot v(s)$. Then show that u and v are inverse functions of each other, hence the name inverse Gaussian (Tweedie 1945).

10. Equation (2.9) of Chap. 2 states that a simple random walk starting at 0 with step probability $p < \frac{1}{2}$ will reach a single barrier at $a > 0$ with probability ϱ^a, where $\varrho = p/(1 - p)$. Use the limiting operations leading to Eq. (4.44) to show that under the conditions expressed in Eq. (4.9), for $p < \frac{1}{2}$ (so that the drift $\mu < 0$), the probability ϱ^a tends to $\exp(\frac{2\mu a}{\sigma^2})$. Use this result to confirm the form of the conditional first-passage time density g^* given in Eq. (4.25) for the case when the drift μ is negative.

11. Consider the sample paths of a freely evolving drift-free Wiener process starting at $x_0 > 0$. We copy each original path and implement a reflecting boundary at $a = 0$ by reflecting all portions of the original path that lie below the line $x = 0$, as if the abscissa were a mirror. Then the mirrored copy of any original path that led to $x > 0$ will still end at the position x. Due to the symmetry of the process, the probability of any original and mirrored path remains the same. In

addition, the mirrored copy of any original path that led to position $-x$ will also end at the position x. Relate this construction to Eq. (4.36).

12. In the scenario with two absorbing barriers, one form of the transition density is given by Eq. (4.59). Show that using only the middle term of $n = 0$, this expansion reduces to Eq. (4.20) for the transition density $f(x, t|a)$ in the scenario with one absorbing barrier.

13. Let $\mathbf{M}_t$ be the maximum level that an unrestricted Wiener process (starting at $x_0 = 0$) reaches during the interval $[0, t]$. Observe the basic relation that $\mathbf{M}_t < a$ if and only if the first-passage time $\mathbf{T}_a$ to the level a is larger than t (cf., Eq. (3.16)). Expressed in terms of the distribution functions of $\mathbf{M}_t$ and $\mathbf{T}_a$, we have $M(a|t) = 1 - G(t|a)$.

    Using this relation and the result of Exercise 8, show that the density $m(a|t)$ of $\mathbf{M}_t$ is

$$m(a|t) = \frac{d}{da}[1 - G(t|a)]$$

$$= 2\exp\left(\frac{2\mu a}{\sigma^2}\right)\left[n(-a|\mu t, \sigma^2 t) - \frac{\mu}{\sigma^2}\,\Phi\left(-\frac{a + \mu t}{\sigma\sqrt{t}}\right)\right]$$

where $n(x|\mu, \sigma^2)$ is the normal density with mean μ and variance σ^2.

14. Using the general relation (sometimes called the "Tail formula") for positive random variables with finite means that $E[\mathbf{T}] = \int_0^\infty [1 - P(\mathbf{T} \leq t)]dt$ to show that the expectation of $\mathbf{M}_t$ is given by

$$E[\mathbf{M}_t] = \int_0^\infty [1 - M(a|t)]\,da = \int_0^\infty G(t|a)\,da$$

$$= \mu t \cdot \Phi\left(\frac{\mu}{\sigma}\sqrt{t}\right) + \sigma\sqrt{\frac{t}{2\pi}}\,\exp\left(-\frac{\mu^2}{2\sigma^2}t\right) + \frac{\sigma^2}{2\mu}\left[2\Phi\left(\frac{\mu}{\sigma}\sqrt{t}\right) - 1\right]$$

    Show that in the limit of $\mu \to 0$, we get the result

$$\lim_{\mu \to 0} E[\mathbf{M}_t] = \sigma\sqrt{\frac{2t}{\pi}}$$

    and relate this to our earlier observations regarding the median of $\mathbf{M}_t$ in Section 3.4.

15. What is the conditional probability $G_t(a|x)$ that an unrestricted Wiener diffusion process starting at $X(0) = 0$ had never crossed the level a during the interval $[0, t]$, given that at time t, the level is $X(t) = x$? Here, the final position x is an arbitrary real, and $a \geq \max(0, x)$. For the specific value of $x = 0$, this construction is called the *Brownian bridge* because every contributing sample path starts and ends at $X(0) = X(t) = 0$, thus bridging the interval in between.

According to the definition of conditional probability, we have that the quantity $P[$ level a not crossed in $[0, t] \mid X(t) = x]$ is equal to

$$\frac{P[\text{ level } a \text{ not crossed in } [0, t] \wedge X(t) = x]}{P[X(t) = x]}$$

The numerator is by definition just equal to the transition density $f(x, t|a)$ in the presence of an absorbing barrier at a, as given by Eq. (4.20). Also, for a Wiener process, the denominator is the normal density Eq. (4.17) for $x_0 = 0$, with mean μt and variance $\sigma^2 t$.

Insert these facts to show that the distribution function $G_t(a|x)$ of the maximum $\mathbf{M}_t$ of the Wiener process in $[0, t]$, conditional on $X(t) = x$, is

$$P[\, \mathbf{M}_t \leq a|X(t) = x\,] \;=\; G_t(a|x) = 1 \;-\; \exp\left[-\frac{2a(a - x)}{\sigma^2 t}\right]$$

for $a \geq \max(0, x)$. Give an intuitive explanation of the remarkable fact that G_t does not depend on μ.

Show that the expected maximum $\mathbf{M}_t$ of the Wiener process in $[0, t]$, given that $X(t) = x$, is

$$E[\mathbf{M}_t|X(t) = x] = \int_0^\infty [1 - G_t(a|x)] \, da$$

$$= \max(0, x) + \sigma \sqrt{\frac{\pi t}{2}} \, \exp\left(\frac{x^2}{2\sigma^2 t}\right) \Phi\left(-\frac{|x|}{\sigma \sqrt{t}}\right)$$

Chapter 5
More General Diffusion Processes

5.1 Diffusion Processes with State-Dependent Drift and Variance

A central characteristic of the Wiener process is that its drift μ and variance σ^2 are independent of the state (position) that the process currently occupies. For example, the displacement of a Wiener process during short time intervals of length Δt will on average be equal to $\mu \Delta t$, independent of the current position of the process. Similarly, the variance of the displacement of a Wiener process during short time intervals does not depend on the current position of the process and equals $\sigma^2 \Delta t$. In some contexts, these assumptions can be too restrictive, and then more flexible models incorporating a possibly state-dependent drift or variance term are more adequate.

The conceptual extensions needed to this end may be understood as natural generalizations of the corresponding assumptions underlying the Wiener process. To this end, let us again consider the mean and variance of the displacement $X(t + \Delta t) - X(t)$ of the process in a small time interval $[t, t + \Delta t]$. For the Wiener process, this mean and variance is simply $\mu \Delta t$ and $\sigma^2 \Delta t$, independent of the current state $X(t) = x$ of the process. To express the notion that the mean and variance of the displacement may possibly vary with the local position x, we write $\mu(x)$ and $\sigma^2(x)$ for the "local" mean and variance of $X(t + \Delta t) - X(t)$.

The more specific constructive interpretation of this notion is as follows. Assume that at time t, the process occupies state $X(t) = x$. Then in the next short time interval $[t, t + \Delta t]$, the displacement $X(t + \Delta t) - X(t)$ will have a mean of $\mu(x)\Delta t$ and variance equal to $\sigma^2(x)\Delta t$. Put more technically, the infinitesimal mean $\mu(x)$ is defined as the limit

$$\mu(x) = \lim_{\Delta t \to 0} \frac{\mathsf{E}[X(t + \Delta t) - X(t)|X(t) = x]}{\Delta t} \tag{5.1}$$

© Springer Nature Switzerland AG 2022
W. Schwarz, *Random Walk and Diffusion Models*,
https://doi.org/10.1007/978-3-031-12100-5_5

and similarly the infinitesimal variance $\sigma^2(x)$ is defined as

$$\sigma^2(x) = \lim_{\Delta t \to 0} \frac{\mathrm{Var}[X(t + \Delta t) - X(t)|X(t) = x]}{\Delta t} \tag{5.2}$$

5.2 The Generalized Forward and Backward Diffusion Equations

How do these more general notions change the nature of the basic framework that we have used so far to analyze diffusion processes? To understand the main conceptual changes implied by state-dependent drift and/or variance terms, we again take up the elementary approach based on Fick's diffusion laws (Sect. 1.2.2). We will once more use the conceptual context of a substance which we imagine to consist of a great number of diffusing particles (cf., Fig. 1.5). As discussed in Sect. 1.2.2, Fick's laws assume that the amount of substance passing through a spatial cross-section in a small time interval $[t, t + \Delta t]$ from left to right at x is proportional i.) to the length, Δt, of the time interval and also ii.) to the gradient (the slope or derivative) of the concentration (or density) f at x at time t.

In Sect. 3.2.2, we saw how these assumptions lead to the basic forward diffusion Equation (3.7). We also considered in Sect. 4.1.2 how this approach generalizes to Eq. (4.12) so as to cover the case of uniform forces (such as gravitation), that is, forces which exert the same strength at any location x. In the present section, we will derive from the Fick assumptions what Marian von Smoluchowski (1915) originally called "the generalized diffusion equation", in which the external force (possibly) varies with the spatial, or state, coordinate x. This case is in fact derived in much the same way as in Sect. 4.1.2, the main difference being that now we have a drift, or force, term equal to $\mu = \mu(x)$. To focus on central ideas, we will (as did von Smoluchowski) for now assume that the diffusion coefficient $D = \frac{1}{2}\sigma^2$ is independent of x. A very similar generalization, summarized below, holds when the variance of the process is state-dependent, too.

In the presence of a force $\mu(x)$ at coordinate x acting into the positive x−direction (i.e., from left to right), the generalized Fick law states that the amount of substance passing in a small time interval $[t, t + \Delta t]$ through a cross-section at x is additively composed of the "pure diffusion" stream, plus the amount of substance passing due to the external force $\mu(x)$.

The assumptions concerning the pure diffusion stream are exactly the same as discussed before in Sect. 3.2.2. That is, this component is negatively proportional to the concentration gradient $\frac{\partial f}{\partial x}$ at x and also proportional to the length Δt of the short time interval considered.

The component of concentration change due to the external force $\mu(x)$ corresponds to ordinary deterministic particle movement as governed by the momentum, that is, by mass $\times$ velocity. More explicitly, the amount of substance passing from left to right through x in a small time interval $[t, t + \Delta t]$ due to the external force is assumed to be proportional (i) to Δt, (ii) to the local concentration f at x and t, and (iii) to the external force acting at x, that is, to $\mu(x)$.

In the analogy to momentum, of the two latter factors, the first, $f(x, t)$, corresponds to mass. The higher (lower) the concentration f at x, the more (less) the substance we expect to pass through a cross-section at x during the interval $[t, t + \Delta t]$. For example, when there is very little substance concentrated at x at time t to begin with, then the force $\mu(x)$ will create only a trickle across a section at x. The third factor, $\mu(x)$, is the local drift rate at x; in the analogy to momentum, it corresponds to velocity. The larger (smaller) the external force at x acting into the positive x-direction, the more (less) the substance we expect to pass through a cross-section.

To summarize the additive contribution of pure diffusion and of the three components just discussed more formally, according to these assumptions, the total amount of substance passing in $[t, t + \Delta t]$ through a cross-section at x will be equal to

$$\left[-\frac{1}{2}\sigma^2 \frac{\partial f}{\partial x} + \mu(x) f(x, t) \right] \Delta t \tag{5.3}$$

As in Sect. 4.1.2, our basic strategy, illustrated in Fig. 3.1, is again to consider first the inflow during Δt at the lower (left) border $x - \Delta x/2$ into the small region $I = [x - \Delta x/2, x + \Delta x/2]$. Next, we obtain the net change by subtracting the flow out of I at the upper (right) border $x + \Delta x/2$. Finally, we simplify the resulting difference of inflow minus outflow that takes place during Δt.

According to Eq. (5.3), there will be a (positive or negative) inflow into I at the left border $x - \Delta x/2$ equal to

$$\text{in} = \left[-\frac{1}{2}\sigma^2 \frac{\partial f(x - \Delta x/2, t)}{\partial x} + \mu(x - \Delta x/2) f(x - \Delta x/2, t) \right] \Delta t$$

Similarly, during the same time interval, there will be a (positive or negative) flow out of I at the right border $x + \Delta x/2$ equal to

$$\text{out} = \left[-\frac{1}{2}\sigma^2 \frac{\partial f(x + \Delta x/2, t)}{\partial x} + \mu(x + \Delta x/2) f(x + \Delta x/2, t) \right] \Delta t$$

As before, all other particles further away from I will not influence the change of the content of I in the small time interval considered. Therefore, the total change of the amount of substance in I in $[t, t + \Delta t]$ will correspond to the difference of inflow minus outflow which, after regrouping the terms, gives

$$\text{in} - \text{out} = \left\{ \frac{1}{2}\sigma^2 \frac{\partial}{\partial x} \left[f(x + \Delta x/2, t) - f(x - \Delta x/2, t) \right] - \right.$$

$$\left. \left[\mu(x + \Delta x/2) f(x + \Delta x/2, t) - \mu(x - \Delta x/2) f(x - \Delta x/2, t) \right] \right\} \Delta t$$

Based on Eq. (3.4), we approximate as usual $f(x + \Delta x/2, t) - f(x - \Delta x/2, t)$
by $\frac{\partial}{\partial x} f(x, t) \Delta x$. In essentially the same manner, we approximate the difference
$\mu(x + \Delta x/2) f(x + \Delta x/2, t) - \mu(x - \Delta x/2) f(x - \Delta x/2, t)$ by the differential
$\frac{\partial}{\partial x} [\mu(x) f(x, t)] \Delta x$ and get

$$\text{in} - \text{out} = \left\{ \frac{1}{2} \sigma^2 \frac{\partial^2}{\partial x^2} f(x, t) - \frac{\partial}{\partial x} [\mu(x) f(x, t)] \right\} \Delta x \Delta t \tag{5.4}$$

On the other hand, the amount of substance in I at time t must be very nearly
equal to $f(x, t) \Delta x$. Correspondingly, the rate of change of this amount in a small
interval $[t, t + \Delta t]$ will tend to $\frac{\partial f(x, t)}{\partial t} \Delta x \Delta t$. Equating this expression for the
change to Eq. (5.4) and then dividing both sides by $\Delta x \Delta t$ give the generalized
forward diffusion equation

$$\frac{\partial f(x, t)}{\partial t} = \frac{1}{2} \sigma^2 \frac{\partial^2}{\partial x^2} f(x, t) - \frac{\partial}{\partial x} [\mu(x) f(x, t)] \tag{5.5}$$

which Marian von Smoluchowski derived in 1915. Again, when $\mu(x) = \mu$, Eq. (5.5)
reduces to Eq. (4.12), as it should, and $\mu(x) = 0$ gives Eq. (3.7).

The case in which the diffusion coefficient $D = \frac{1}{2} \sigma^2$ is state-dependent is
handled in much the same manner. As before, we assume that at time t, the purely
diffusive stream at x is proportional to the concentration gradient $\frac{\partial f}{\partial x}$ at x and to the
length of the (short) time interval Δt considered. The only change required is that
the factor of proportionality may itself change with x. As this change concerns only
the first component $-\frac{1}{2} \sigma^2 \frac{\partial f}{\partial x}$ that appears in Eq. (5.3), this modification clearly
leads to the generalized forward diffusion equation

$$\frac{\partial f(x_0, x, t)}{\partial t} = \frac{1}{2} \frac{\partial^2}{\partial x^2} [\sigma^2(x) f(x_0, x, t)] - \frac{\partial}{\partial x} [\mu(x) f(x_0, x, t)] \tag{5.6}$$

where we have added the starting position $X(0) = x_0$ to our notation to make more
explicit that the density f evidently also depends on x_0. Specifically, the above
arguments show that Eq. (5.6) must hold in x and t for any arbitrary, fixed value of
x_0.

The forward diffusion Equation (5.6) relates changes in t to those in the state
variable x; it holds for any given, fixed starting point x_0. We have seen in Sect. 4.1.3
that the forward Equation (4.12) for the Wiener process is complemented by the
corresponding backward Equation (4.16) which relates changes in t to those in
the starting point x_0, for any given, fixed state variable x. We thus expect that a
backward equation corresponding to the general forward diffusion Equation (5.6)
holds as well. Generalizing the basic approach described in Sect. 4.1.3 by the same
technique that we used above to derive Eq. (5.5), it may indeed be shown that the

generalized backward equation in t and x_0

$$\frac{\partial f(x_0, x, t)}{\partial t} = \frac{1}{2}\sigma^2(x_0)\frac{\partial^2}{\partial x_0^2} f(x_0, x, t) + \mu(x_0)\frac{\partial}{\partial x_0} f(x_0, x, t) \qquad (5.7)$$

holds for any given, fixed x. Note that for $\mu(x_0) = \mu$ and $\sigma^2(x_0) = \sigma^2$, the general backward Equation (5.7) reduces to Eq. (4.16) which holds for the Wiener process.

One important usage of Eq. (5.7) is in situations with an absorbing barrier at $x = a > x_0$. Similar to our approach in Sect. 4.2.2 for the Wiener process, we define $F(x_0, x, t)$ to be the probability for a diffusion process starting at x_0 not to have reached the barrier a during $[0, t]$ and to be below the level x at time t. We consider the process during a small time interval at some state x below the barrier a. The local dynamics at x is governed by the infinitesimal mean $\mu(x)$ and variance $\sigma^2(x)$, which as we saw leads to the generalized backward Equation (5.7) for the corresponding density $f(x_0, x, t) = \frac{\partial}{\partial x}F(x_0, x, t)$. Integrating Eq. (5.7) over x, this implies that $F(x_0, x, t)$ will also satisfy Eq. (5.7), for fixed values of the state variable x. Looking, specifically, at the value of $x = a$, the function $F(x_0, a, t)$ represents the survivor function of the first-passage time T_a from x_0 to $x = a$, and so $-\frac{\partial}{\partial t}F(x_0, a, t)$ is the first-passage time density $g(t|a, x_0)$. Given that $F(x_0, x, t)$ satisfies Eq. (5.7) in the variables x_0 and t, the function $-\frac{\partial}{\partial t}F(x_0, a, t)$, and therefore $g(t|a, x_0)$, will satisfy this equation in x_0 and t, too. In summary, then, we find that in a diffusion process with infinitesimal mean $\mu(x)$ and variance $\sigma^2(x)$, the density $g(t|a, x_0)$ of the first-passage time T_a from x_0 to a will satisfy

$$\frac{\partial g(t|a, x_0)}{\partial t} = \frac{1}{2}\sigma^2(x_0) \cdot \frac{\partial^2 g(t|a, x_0)}{\partial x_0^2} + \mu(x_0) \cdot \frac{\partial g(t|a, x_0)}{\partial x_0} \qquad (5.8)$$

In many cases, Eq. (5.8) is difficult to solve explicitly, and one must resort to numerical solutions (e.g., Smith 1985). However, in Chap. 6, we will see that Eq. (5.8) forms the basis to obtain information at least about absorption probabilities and means of first-passage times of generalized diffusion processes in a systematic and fairly direct manner.

5.3 Examples of More General Diffusion Processes

In this section, we consider two important examples to illustrate the general notions of the preceding sections.

Our first example describes the Ornstein–Uhlenbeck,[1] for short: OU, process. This example covers the case in which $\mu(x)$ is (linearly) dependent on x, whereas $\sigma^2(x)$ is constant. In many aspects, it represents the continuous counterpart of the discrete Ehrenfest model treated in detail in Sect. 2.5.1.

Our second example, the Fisher–Wright process of random genetic drift, is the continuous counterpart of the discrete Fisher–Wright model of Sect. 2.5.2. It describes the dynamic changes in the proportion of allele$-a$ individuals in a given population when the genetic replacement from generation to generation is purely random (the basic qualitative ideas motivating this model are explained in Sect. 2.5.2). Whereas in the OU process $\mu(x)$ depends on x and $\sigma^2(x)$ is constant, for the Fisher–Wright process, the infinitesimal mean $\mu(x)$ is constant (in fact, equal to zero) but $\sigma^2(x)$ varies with x.

5.3.1   The Ornstein–Uhlenbeck (OU) Process

As noted above, in some contexts, the assumption underlying the Wiener process of a state-independent drift term seems too restrictive. As an alternative, the OU process is defined by having, specifically, a *linear* state-dependent drift, which in the following we will writè in the form

$$\mu(x) = \mu - kx \tag{5.9}$$

while keeping the assumption of the Wiener process that $\sigma^2(x) = \sigma^2$.

Here, μ is a constant drift component that may take any real value, as in a Wiener process. If positive, the parameter k describes a *restoring force* which results, in addition to the constant drift component μ, in a downward drift component for positive states, $x > 0$, and in an upward drift component for negative states, $x < 0$. Processes with this characteristic are often called *mean-reverting*. This dynamic is reminiscent of the discrete Ehrenfest model described in Sect. 2.5.1 in that large excursions from intermediate states increase the probability of reverting moves. Intuitively, we then expect the build-up of a stationary distribution after the process has been in operation for a long time.

On the other hand, if the parameter k is negative, then the term $-kx$ represents a *repelling force*. In this case, large excursions are, with high probability, followed by even larger excursions into the same direction. Evidently, if $k = 0$, then $\mu(x) = \mu$, and the OU process then simplifies to a Wiener process with drift μ as a special case.

If $\mu = 0$, then for $k > 0$, the OU process will generally tend to $x = 0$, having a negative (positive) drift $\mu(x)$ for positive (negative) states. A physical analogy

---

[1] After the physicists L.S. Ornstein and G.E. Uhlenbeck who in 1930 described central properties of this model.

of this case is Hooke's law, when the states $X(t)$ refer to the (positive or negative) deflection of a spring at time t and $x = 0$ represents a balanced equilibrium state. According to Hooke's law, the restoring force $\mu(x)$ back to the equilibrium point of the spring is negatively proportional to its current deflection, corresponding to $\mu(x) = -kx$.

To gain more insight into the OU process, we start from two elementary facts. First, we know from Eq. (4.17) that the transition density of a Wiener process is given by

$$f(x_0, x, t) = \frac{1}{\sigma\sqrt{2\pi t}} \exp\left[-\frac{(x - x_0 - \mu t)^2}{2\sigma^2 t} \right] \tag{5.10}$$

where as usual μ is the drift, σ^2 the variance, and x_0 the starting point of the Wiener process at $t = 0$.

Second, according to the so-called renewal (or Chapman-Kolmogorov) equation, we must have

$$f(x_0, y, t) = \int_{-\infty}^{\infty} f(x_0, x, \tau) \cdot f(x, y, t - \tau)\, dx \tag{5.11}$$

Equation (5.11) rests on a simple but powerful insight that holds for any stationary Markovian process, not just the Wiener process. The left-hand side of Eq. (5.11) is the density for a process to be at time t at position (or state) y, when at $t = 0$ it started at x_0. At the fixed intermediate time $0 < \tau < t$, this process must then have been at *some* position (let us call it x) and then from there on have reached state y in the remaining time $t - \tau$. Integrating across all possible values of the intermediate state x exhausts all possible paths leading from x_0 to y, and we get Eq. (5.11). Note that Eq. (5.11) rests on the Markovian property because it assumes that the path leading from x to y in $[\tau, t]$ is independent of the way in which the process had reached x from x_0 in $[0, \tau]$. It is only on this Markovian basis that we may factor the densities appearing in the integrand of Eq. (5.11). Note also that our notation assumes stationary increments: the density for a displacement from x_0 to y depends only on the length of the interval t, but not on the absolute location on the time axis.

We now consider a OU process $X(t)$ starting at x_0, with a local (i.e., state-dependent) drift rate $\mu(x) = \mu - kx$ and variance parameter σ^2. Roughly speaking, this means that when $X(t) = x$, then during a short time interval of length Δt, the displacement $X(t+\Delta t) - X(t)$ will on average be equal to $\mu(x)\Delta t$, and the variance of the displacement will be $\sigma^2 \Delta t$.

Let us first focus on the short interval $[0, \Delta t]$, where for now Δt is considered a small but finite duration; as always, we proceed with a view to study eventually the limit as $\Delta t \to 0$. As long as Δt is small, $X(t)$ will not move away a great distance from x_0 in $[0, \Delta t]$, and for this reason, the actual state-dependent drift $\mu(x)$ at any point during this interval cannot be very different from $\mu(x_0) = \mu - kx_0$. The error in this approximation will decrease in Δt and will tend to zero as $\Delta t \to 0$. In effect, then, we approximate the *state-dependent* drift $\mu(x)$ by the *constant* drift $\mu(x_0)$

during the short interval $[0, \Delta t]$. Within this approximation, according to Eq. (5.10), the density f for states of X at time $t = \Delta t$ would clearly be normal, with mean $x_0 + (\mu - kx_0)\Delta t$ and variance $\sigma^2 \Delta t$. Therefore,

$$\mathsf{E}[X(\Delta t)] = x_0 + (\mu - kx_0)\Delta t = \lambda x_0 + \mu \Delta t$$

$$\mathsf{Var}[X(\Delta t)] = \sigma^2 \Delta t$$

where $\lambda = 1 - k\Delta t$. Note that $\lambda > 0$, as Δt is small. When $k = 0$, then $\lambda = 1$, and the OU process simplifies to the Wiener process.

We next consider the density f at time $t = 2\Delta t$ and use the renewal Eq. (5.11), specifically, with $\tau = \Delta t$ and $t = 2\Delta t$. We already know that for small Δt $f(x_0, x, \Delta t)$ tends to a normal density, with mean $\lambda x_0 + \mu \Delta t$ and variance $\sigma^2 \Delta t$. We then approximate the second factor of the integrand in Eq. (5.11), regarding the displacement in $[\Delta t, 2\Delta t]$: given that $X(\Delta t) = x$, the random variable $X(2\Delta t)$ is again nearly normal, with mean $x + (\mu - kx)\Delta t = \lambda x + \mu \Delta t$ and variance $\sigma^2 \Delta t$. The logic here is much the same as before, regarding the interval $[0, \Delta t]$, with the exception that the "start point" (at $t = \Delta t$) on which we condition now is the random position $X(\Delta t) = x$ rather than the fixed starting position x_0. According to the renewal Eq. (5.11), we then integrate across the possible positions $X(\Delta t) = x$ and get

$$f(x_0, y, 2\Delta t) = \int_{-\infty}^{\infty} \frac{1}{\sigma\sqrt{2\pi \Delta t}} \exp\left[-\frac{1}{2\sigma^2 \Delta t}(x - \lambda x_0 - \mu \Delta t)^2 \right]$$

$$\cdot \frac{1}{\sigma\sqrt{2\pi \Delta t}} \exp\left[-\frac{1}{2\sigma^2 \Delta t}(y - \lambda x - \mu \Delta t)^2 \right] dx$$

By elementary algebra, the integral may be shown to be another normal density, with mean and variance

$$\mathsf{E}[X(2\Delta t)] = \lambda^2 x_0 + \mu \Delta t(1 + \lambda)$$

$$\mathsf{Var}[X(2\Delta t)] = \sigma^2 \Delta t (1 + \lambda^2)$$

Note that when $k > 0$, we have $0 < \lambda < 1$ which implies that the variance is smaller than for the Wiener process which corresponds to the case $k = 0$ giving $\lambda = 1$ and for which the variance equals $2\sigma^2 \Delta t$.

These results suggest a clear pattern. Based on Eq. (5.11), we might now continue with the same arguments and would find that for general n, using well-known summation formulae, and the relation $1 - \lambda = k\Delta t$

$$\mathsf{E}[X(n\Delta t)] = \lambda^n x_0 + \mu \Delta t \sum_{i=0}^{n-1} \lambda^i$$

$$= \lambda^n x_0 + \mu \Delta t \frac{1 - \lambda^n}{1 - \lambda}$$

$$= \lambda^n \left(x_0 - \frac{\mu}{k} \right) + \frac{\mu}{k} \tag{5.12}$$

$$\text{Var}[X(n\Delta t)] = \sigma^2 \Delta t \sum_{i=0}^{n-1} \lambda^{2i}$$

$$= \sigma^2 \Delta t \, \frac{1 - \lambda^{2n}}{1 - \lambda^2} \tag{5.13}$$

The above construction of analyzing successive Δt−intervals (originally due to von Smoluchowski, 1913) is highly instructive as regards the dynamics underlying the OU process. However, the final results Eqs. (5.12) and (5.13) are found much easier from the standard relations regarding conditional expectation and conditional variance that we had used before in Sects. 2.4.4 and 2.5, as follows.

Given the state $X(n\Delta t)$ of the process at time $n\Delta t$, the displacement of the OU process during the next short time interval of length Δt will on average be equal to $[\mu - kX(n\Delta t)]\Delta t$. We therefore get the recursive relation

$$\text{E}[X((n+1)\Delta t)] = \text{E}[\text{E}[X((n+1)\Delta t)|X(n\Delta t)]]$$

$$= \text{E}[X(n\Delta t) + [\mu - kX(n\Delta t)]\Delta t]$$

$$= \text{E}[(1 - k\Delta t)X(n\Delta t) + \mu\Delta t]$$

$$= \lambda \, \text{E}[X(n\Delta t)] + \mu\Delta t \tag{5.14}$$

which, starting from $\text{E}[X(\Delta t)] = \lambda x_0 + \mu\Delta t$ (i.e., the case $n = 1$ that we considered in detail above), clearly leads to Eq. (5.12).

Similarly, according to the conditional variance formula discussed in Sect. 2.4.4,

$$\text{Var}[X((n+1)\Delta t)] =$$

$$\text{E}[\text{Var}[X((n+1)\Delta t)|X(n\Delta t)]] + \text{Var}[\text{E}[X((n+1)\Delta t)|X(n\Delta t)]] \tag{5.15}$$

The inner variance expression $\text{Var}[X((n+1)\Delta t)|X(n\Delta t)]$ in the first term on the right-hand side of Eq. (5.15) clearly equals $\sigma^2\Delta t$, the state-independent variance of the displacement of the OU process in an interval of length Δt. We also noted above that the inner expectation in the second term on the right-hand side of Eq. (5.15), $\text{E}[X((n+1)\Delta t)|X(n\Delta t)]$, equals $\lambda \, X(n\Delta t) + \mu\Delta t$, the expected displacement in an interval of length Δt, added to the given position $X(n\Delta t)$ at start. Inserting these partial results, we get the recursive relation

$$\text{Var}[X((n+1)\Delta t)] = \text{E}[\sigma^2\Delta t] + \text{Var}[\lambda \, X(n\Delta t) + \mu\Delta t]$$

$$= \sigma^2\Delta t + \lambda^2 \, \text{Var}[\, X(n\Delta t)] \tag{5.16}$$

which, starting from $\text{Var}[X(\Delta t)] = \sigma^2\Delta t$, leads to our previous variance result in Eq. (5.13).

It is now easy to find from Eqs. (5.12) and (5.13) the limits of these expressions for $\Delta t \to 0$, for which the error of our discrete approximation will tend to zero. To this end, we look at a fixed time $t = n\Delta t$ and then let $n \to \infty$ and $\Delta t \to 0$ such that t remains fixed. This corresponds to our usual limiting procedure to partition the given interval $[0, t]$ into increasingly more (n) subintervals of decreasing duration (Δt) and produces, with $\Delta t = t/n$, the limit

$$\lambda^n = (1 - k\Delta t)^n = (1 - kt/n)^n \to \exp(-kt)$$

and thus from Eq. (5.12) for the expected position of the OU process at time t

$$\mathsf{E}[X(t)] = \exp(-kt)\left(x_0 - \frac{\mu}{k}\right) + \frac{\mu}{k} \tag{5.17}$$

Equation (5.17) represents a continuous counterpart to Eq. (2.57) for the discrete Ehrenfest model. The variance parameter σ^2 has no influence on $\mathsf{E}[X(t)]$, as in the Wiener process. As expected, for $k > 0$, the OU process tends in the limit of large t to a stationary average level, equal to μ/k. The sign of this level then depends on the sign of μ and its absolute value on the magnitude of the constant drift component μ relative to the restoring force k. The stationary mean μ/k may be interpreted as an equilibrium, or a compromise, between the drift μ which drives the process away from zero and the restoring force $k > 0$ which has the opposite effect. It is not difficult to show from Eq. (5.17) that as $k \to 0$, we get $\mathsf{E}[X(t)] \to x_0 + \mu t$, as expected for the limiting case of a Wiener process.

To obtain the corresponding variance result in continuous time from Eq. (5.13), we first note that, again using the relation $\Delta t = t/n$,

$$\lambda^{2n} = (1 - k\Delta t)^{2n} = (1 - \frac{2kt}{2n})^{2n} \to \exp(-2kt)$$

so that $1 - \lambda^{2n}$ tends to $1 - \exp(-2kt)$.

We also see that the remaining expression in Eq. (5.13)

$$\frac{\sigma^2 \Delta t}{1 - \lambda^2} = \frac{\sigma^2 \Delta t}{1 - (1 - 2k\Delta t + k^2(\Delta t)^2)} = \frac{\sigma^2 t/n}{2kt/n - k^2 t^2/n^2}$$

$$= \frac{\sigma^2}{2k - k^2 t/n} \to \frac{\sigma^2}{2k} \quad , \text{ as } n \to \infty .$$

Together, then, by Eq. (5.13), the variance of the OU process at time t is

$$\mathsf{Var}[X(t)] = \frac{\sigma^2}{2k}\left[1 - \exp(-2kt)\right] \tag{5.18}$$

Again, as $k \rightarrow 0$, we get $\mathsf{Var}[X(t)] \rightarrow \sigma^2 t$, the result known from the Wiener process. Note that, just as in the Wiener process, the constant drift component μ and the starting value x_0 have no influence on $\mathsf{Var}[X(t)]$.

In summary, $X(t)$ is for all t normally distributed, with a mean given by Eq. (5.17) and variance given by Eq. (5.18). If $k > 0$, then the term $-kx$ in Eq. (5.9) for $\mu(x)$ represents a restoring force producing an equilibrium in which for large t the stationary normal distribution of $X(t)$ has mean μ/k and variance $\sigma^2/(2k)$.

The results Eqs. (5.17) and (5.18) remain valid in the case of $k < 0$, when the force is repelling rather than restoring. However, in this case, no stationary density exists, as is clear from the construction of the process. It is only for positive values of k that large excursions into one direction make it increasingly likely that "compensating steps" into the other direction will follow; for negative values of k, the process will tend to increasingly large excursions. As indicated by Eq. (5.17), for negative values of k, the OU process tends to $+\infty$ if the process starts at $x_0 > \mu/k$ and to $-\infty$ if the start point $x_0 < \mu/k$.

5.3.2 The Fisher–Wright Process

In Sect. 2.5.2, we described the discrete Fisher–Wright model in which the number of individuals carrying an $a-$allele in successive generations is described by a mechanism of binomial sampling of alleles. As we discussed at the end of Sect. 2.5.2, a convenient standardized representation of the Fisher–Wright model is to look at the associated process defined by the relative proportion of allele$-a$ individuals. The analysis of the discrete model suggested to us that the mean displacement in any small time interval (corresponding conceptually to one generation) in this proportion process will be zero and that the variance of this displacement, given the current proportion is equal to x, will be $x(1-x)/m$, where m corresponds to the size of the population (cf., Eq. (2.66)). This conceptual background forms a main motivation to study the corresponding Fisher–Wright diffusion process in continuous time in which the infinitesimal mean and variance are given as

$$\mu(x) = 0 \qquad \text{and} \qquad \sigma^2(x) = kx(1-x) \tag{5.19}$$

respectively.

We define the state variable $0 \leq X(t) \leq 1$ of this process as the relative proportion of allele$-a$ individuals at time t and denote as x_0 the initial proportion at time $t = 0$. Let us first determine the mean value of $X(t)$ for this process as a function of t. To this end, we use the basic properties governing the Fisher–Wright process and seek to relate $\mathsf{E}[X(t + \Delta t)]$ to $\mathsf{E}[X(t)]$. More specifically, to find $\mathsf{E}[X(t + \Delta t)]$, we first condition on the value of $X(t)$ and then express

$E[X(t + \Delta t)]$ in terms of $X(t)$. Formally, using conditional expectation much as we did in Eq. (2.61)

$$E[X(t + \Delta t)] = E[E[X(t + \Delta t)|X(t)]] \tag{5.20}$$

Now, $X(t + \Delta t)$ may be represented by the two independent additive components $[X(t + \Delta t) - X(t)] + X(t)$. The first part $X(t + \Delta t) - X(t)$ represents the displacement of the process in the interval $[t, t + \Delta t]$. Given $X(t)$, for small Δt, the mean of this displacement is $\mu[X(t)] \Delta t = 0$ because $\mu(x) = 0$ in the Fisher–Wright process. Therefore,

$$E[X(t + \Delta t)] = E[0 + X(t)] = E[X(t)] \tag{5.21}$$

which corresponds closely to Eq. (2.61) for the discrete version of the model. Formally, we may subtract $E[X(t)]$ on both sides of Eq. (5.21) and divide by Δt, then forming the limit of $\Delta t \to 0$. This approach shows that $\frac{d}{dt} E[X(t)] = 0$, so that $E[X(t)]$ is at most a constant. Given that initially $X(0) = x_0$, we must then have that $E[X(t)] = x_0$, exactly as in the discrete counterpart analyzed in Sect. 2.5.2.

To derive $\text{Var}[X(t)]$, we again (cf., Eq. (5.15)) use the conditional variance formula, in a form which is the direct counterpart to Eq. (2.62) used for the discrete version of the Fisher–Wright model,

$$\text{Var}[X(t + \Delta t)] = E[\text{Var}[X(t + \Delta t)|X(t)]] + \text{Var}[E[X(t + \Delta t)|X(t)]] \tag{5.22}$$

Let us inspect the two summands on the right-hand side of Eq. (5.22) in turn. Note that the inner variance expression $\text{Var}[X(t + \Delta t)|X(t)]$ in the first term might as well be written as $\text{Var}[X(t + \Delta t) - X(t)|X(t)]$. The reason is that adding or subtracting a constant does not affect the variance; conditioning on $X(t)$, this variable acts as a constant regarding the (conditional) variance of $X(t + \Delta t)$. Now, $X(t + \Delta t) - X(t)$ is the displacement of the process in the interval $[t, t + \Delta t]$; given $X(t)$, for small Δt, its (conditional) variance is equal to $\sigma^2[X(t)] \Delta t = kX(t)[1 - X(t)] \Delta t$. Therefore, using the fact derived from Eq. (5.21) that $E[X(t)] = x_0$, the first term on the right-hand side of Eq. (5.22) equals

$$\begin{aligned}
E[\text{Var}[X(t + \Delta t)|X(t)]] &= E[kX(t)[1 - X(t)]\Delta t] \\
&= k \left\{ E[X(t)] - E[X^2(t)] \right\} \Delta t \\
&= k \left\{ E[X(t)] - \text{Var}[X(t)] - E^2[X(t)] \right\} \Delta t \\
&= -k \, \text{Var}[X(t)] \, \Delta t + k \, x_0(1 - x_0) \, \Delta t
\end{aligned}$$

The inner conditional expectation $E[X(t + \Delta t)|X(t)]$ in the second summand on the right-hand side Eq. (5.22) is clearly just equal to $X(t)$, as on average the process does not change in $[t, t + \Delta t]$. Together, then, we may write Eq. (5.22) in the form

$$\text{Var}[X(t + \Delta t)] = -k\,\text{Var}[X(t)]\,\Delta t + k\,x_0(1 - x_0)\,\Delta t + \text{Var}[X(t)] \quad (5.23)$$

We subtract $\text{Var}[X(t)]$ on both sides of Eq. (5.23), then divide by Δt, and form as usual the limit $\Delta t \to 0$, to get a first-order differential equation for $\text{Var}[X(t)]$

$$\frac{d}{dt}\,\text{Var}[X(t)] = -k\,\text{Var}[X(t)] + k\,x_0(1 - x_0) \quad (5.24)$$

The solution of Eq. (5.24) satisfying $\text{Var}[X(0)] = 0$ is

$$\text{Var}[X(t)] = x_0(1 - x_0)\,[\,1 - \exp(-kt)\,] \quad (5.25)$$

For large t, the expression for $\text{Var}[X(t)]$ increases toward $x_0(1 - x_0)$. As expected, the result Eq. (5.25) corresponds directly to the related variance result Eq. (2.64) for the discrete version of the Fisher–Wright model. At $t = 0$, the state is fixed by the initial condition, and so the variance is zero. In the long run, $X(t)$ will either equal 1 or 0, with probabilities x_0 and $1 - x_0$, respectively, producing the asymptotic variance.

5.4 Siegert's Equation for First-Passage Times

In the preceding sections, we have seen that diffusion processes more general than the Wiener process can be characterized by their infinitesimal mean and variance, $\mu(x)$ and $\sigma^2(x)$. Our description so far referred to the unrestricted evolution of these corresponding diffusion processes, when absorbing or reflecting barriers are absent. It seems intuitively clear that the transition density of the unrestricted process, together with initial and boundary conditions, must in some way also determine the first-passage time densities associated with this process (cf., Sect. 4.2). In this section, we consider a basic result on first-passage times for general diffusion processes originally due to Siegert (1951). It describes a general relation between the transition density of an unrestricted diffusion process and the density of its first-passage time through a given level a. In the next section, we then apply and illustrate this general result for the special case of the Wiener process.

In many cases, the transition density is the primary description available for a given diffusion process, for example, as a solution of Eqs. (5.6) or (5.7). Siegert's equation assumes that the diffusion process is continuous and that it has independent and stationary displacements; the latter property means that the transition density $P[X(s + t) = y | X(s) = x]$ depends only on the temporal separation t, but does not change with s. Therefore, much as we did in Eq. (5.11), we can write this transition density for the unrestricted process more simply as $P(y, t | x)$, the density to be at position y when t time units before it was at position x. For example, if we study a

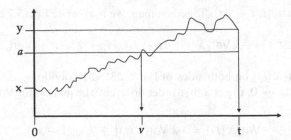

Fig. 5.1 Abscissa, time t; ordinate, spatial position of the path starting at x and ending at y. Any continuous path leading from $(0|x)$ to $(t|y)$ must at some point $0 < v < t$ reach the intermediate level a (where $x < a < y$) for the first time. The density of the time v when this level a is reached first is $g(v|a, x)$. Also, the transition density of moving (not necessarily for the first time) to the level y from a in the remaining time $t - v$ is by definition given as $P(y, t - v|a)$. The overall transition density to be at level y at time t when starting (at time 0) at level x is the sum (integral) across all corresponding sample path combinations with different values of v

Wiener process with drift μ starting at x, then the process is characterized by the fact that $P(y, t|x)$ is a normal density for the variable y with mean $x + \mu t$ and variance $\sigma^2 t$.

Siegert's equation rests on an elementary but powerful property, originally noted by Schrödinger (1915), that is illustrated in Fig. 5.1. In fact, the argument is quite similar to the reasoning leading to the renewal Equation (5.11). We consider a diffusion process starting at x and denote as $P(y, t|x)$ the stationary transition density for it to be at time t at level $y > x$, not necessarily for the first time, of course. Consider a level a that is intermediate between x and y, that is, $x < a < y$. Now, a continuous process starting at x that at time t is at the level $y > x$ must necessarily have reached the intermediate level a *for the first time* at some intermediate time v in $[0, t]$. That is, the total transition from $X(0) = x$ to $X(t) = y$ can be additively decomposed into an epoch $[0, v]$ until the process starting from x reaches a for the first time, plus an additional epoch $[v, t]$ in which it then moves from a to y. The first epoch is by definition just the first-passage time from x to a. The condition for the second epoch means that in the remaining interval $[v, t]$, the process makes a transition from a to y. For a process with independent, stationary displacements, the latter transition has the density $P(y, t - v|a)$. If we denote (as we did in Eq. (4.24)) the density of the first-passage time v from x to a as $g(v|a, x)$, then integrating across all possible values of $0 < v < t$, we have the integral equation

$$P(y, t|x) = \int_0^t g(v|a, x) \cdot P(y, t - v|a)\, dv \qquad (5.26)$$

Equation (5.26) implicitly defines a relation between the transition density, P, and the first-passage time density, g. Specifically, for any process with independent, stationary displacements and a given transition density P, we can, in principle, use Eq. (5.26) to find the corresponding first-passage time density g.

The qualification "in principle" in the last sentence means that the form of Eq. (5.26) for the relation of P to g is often not immediately useful in practice. To get a more useful representation, note that Eq. (5.26) is a convolution integral in the time variable. Thus, we use Laplace transforms (with respect to the time variable) to turn the convolution in Eq. (5.26) into a multiplication of the corresponding transforms,

$$\mathsf{P}_L(y, \lambda|x) = g_L(\lambda|a, x) \cdot \mathsf{P}_L(y, \lambda|a) \qquad \text{, that is,}$$

$$g_L(\lambda|a, x) = \frac{\mathsf{P}_L(y, \lambda|x)}{\mathsf{P}_L(y, \lambda|a)} \tag{5.27}$$

where the subscript L indicates the Laplace transform of the indexed function (g or P) and λ is the dummy argument of the Laplace transform. In principle, for any given transition density P, we may first compute its transform P_L and then use Eq. (5.27) to find (the Laplace transform of) the first-passage time density g.

Note that the numerator on the right-hand side of Eq. (5.27) refers (in state space) to the distance $y - x$ and the denominator to the distance $y - a$. Siegert's Equation (5.27) at first appears as a purely formal (if quite general) relation; however, a more intuitive interpretation of its meaning is as follows. In the operational calculus, the *division* of transforms translates back into *differences* (i.e., distances) in state space. Just as common transform *factors* in Eq. (5.27) cancel, so common *distances* in state space are subtracted out. Therefore, the quotient on the right-hand side of Eq. (5.27) refers, independent of y, to the difference of distances in the state space, $(y - x) - (y - a) = a - x$, which is just the to-be-covered distance to which the first-passage time with density g refers.

5.4.1 Application of Siegert's Equation to the Wiener Process

We illustrate Siegert's Equation (5.27) for the case of the Wiener process with drift $\mu > 0$. In the Wiener process, the displacement during any interval of length t is normally distributed, with mean μt and variance $\sigma^2 t$. Therefore, P($y, t|z$) is a normal density with mean $z + \mu t$ and variance $\sigma^2 t$. Note that the Laplace transforms in Eq. (5.27) must be taken with respect to the time variable t, not to the variable y which denotes the value of the state variable that is normally distributed. For any start point z (in the sequel, we will use $z = x$ and $z = a$ in turn), the Laplace transform of P($y, t|z$) is the standard integral (e.g., Abramowitz and Stegun 1965, ch. 29).

$$\mathsf{P}_L(y, \lambda|z) = \int_0^\infty \exp(-\lambda t)\, n(y|z + \mu t, \sigma^2 t)\, dt$$

$$= \frac{1}{\sqrt{(2\lambda\sigma^2 + \mu^2)}} \exp\left[\frac{y - z}{\sigma^2}\left(\mu - \sqrt{2\lambda\sigma^2 + \mu^2}\right)\right]$$

According to Eq. (5.27), $g_L(\lambda|a, x)$ is equal to the ratio of these expressions with starting points $z = x$ (the numerator in Eq. (5.27)) and $z = a$ (the denominator in Eq. (5.27)). Canceling all common factors which depend only on y, λ, μ, and σ (but not on z), we get

$$g_L(\lambda|a, x) = \exp\left[\frac{a-x}{\sigma^2}\left(\mu - \sqrt{2\lambda\sigma^2 + \mu^2}\right)\right] \tag{5.28}$$

This is the Laplace transform of the first-passage time density $g(t|a, x)$ through the level a, starting at $t = 0$ at the level x that we had found before in Eq. (4.34) via a limiting process from the simple random walk.

5.5 The Darling and Siegert Equations

Siegert's Equation (5.27) regarding the first-passage time to a single barrier a is powerful and general, but many applied models require an analysis involving two rather than one absorbing barrier. From a more practical view, it also often proves difficult to find the explicit form of the Laplace transform of the transition density characterizing a specific diffusion process. However, in order to apply Siegert's Eq. (5.27), it is evidently necessary to know the exact form of P_L.

To address these theoretical and practical limitations, the following set of equations, essentially due to Darling and Siegert (1953), is of direct relevance. In essence, the Darling and Siegert equations will permit us to derive basic information about the absorption probabilities and mean first-passage times for general diffusion processes involving one or two absorbing or reflecting barriers under fairly flexible conditions. In this section, we will present the main conceptual approach and some basic results, such as Eq. (5.39). The general framework is then described and applied to specific examples more systematically in Chap. 6.

We consider a diffusion process between two absorbing barriers at $-b$ and a that is characterized by the infinitesimal mean $\mu(x)$ and the infinitesimal variance $\sigma^2(x)$. Our starting point is the fact that the density $g(t|x_0)$ of the first-passage time to either one of the absorbing barriers, no matter which, satisfies the backward Eq. (5.8) (or, for the Wiener process, the simpler corresponding Eq. (4.30))

$$\frac{\partial g(t|x_0)}{\partial t} = \frac{1}{2}\sigma^2(x_0) \cdot \frac{\partial^2 g(t|x_0)}{\partial x_0^2} + \mu(x_0) \cdot \frac{\partial g(t|x_0)}{\partial x_0} \tag{5.29}$$

in the time variable t and the start variable $X(0) = x_0$.

We can think of multiplying both sides of Eq. (5.29) by e^{-st} and then integrating with respect to t over the positive reals. Formally, this procedure corresponds to taking the Laplace transform on both sides of Eq. (5.29). The density $g(t|x_0)$ must vanish at $t = 0$ and converge to zero for large t; therefore, by standard rules (for a detailed exposition, see Wylie and Barrett 1995, ch. 11.8), the Laplace transform of the left-hand side of Eq. (5.29) simplifies to $su(x_0)$ where

$$u(x_0) = \int_0^\infty e^{-st} g(t|x_0)\, dt \qquad (5.30)$$

is the Laplace transform of the first-passage time density $g(t|x_0)$. Of course, $u(x_0)$ also depends on the dummy variable s, but to keep our notation parsimonious and to focus on the central points, we suppress this variable in our notation for u.

To handle the Laplace transform of the right-hand side of Eq. (5.29), we formally interchange the order of integration with respect to t and differentiation with respect to x_0. We also note that the functions $\mu(x_0)$ and $\sigma^2(x_0)$ are independent of t and thus are simply a constant factor as far as the integration with respect to t is concerned. In this way, we get the transformed version of Eq. (5.29)

$$s\, u(x_0) = \frac{1}{2}\sigma^2(x_0)\, u''(x_0) + \mu(x_0)\, u'(x_0) \qquad (5.31)$$

where the function u is as defined in Eq. (5.30) and the primes indicate its differentiation with respect to x_0.

We next use the standard series expansion $e^{-st} = \sum_{i=0}^\infty (-st)^i/i!$ of the exponential function to rewrite the Laplace transform $u(x_0)$ formally as a power series in the variable s, as follows:

$$u(x_0) = \int_0^\infty e^{-st} g(t|x_0)\, dt = \int_0^\infty \left(\sum_{i=0}^\infty \frac{(-st)^i}{i!} \right) g(t|x_0)\, dt$$

$$= \sum_{i=0}^\infty \frac{(-s)^i}{i!} \int_0^\infty t^i\, g(t|x_0)\, dt$$

$$= \sum_{i=0}^\infty \frac{(-s)^i}{i!} m_i(x_0) \qquad (5.32)$$

after interchanging summation and integration.

The expressions $\int_0^\infty t^i g(t|x_0)\, dt$ which appear in the representation of $u(x_0)$ in the second line of Eq. (5.32) represent the i–th moments of the first-passage time for which in the following we write for short $m_i(x_0)$, to emphasize their dependence on the starting point x_0. For example, $m_1(x_0)$ is the mean first-passage time, considered as a function of the starting point x_0. Formally, as $t^0 = 1$, the term corresponding to $i = 0$ is just the integral of $g(t|x_0)$ with respect to t; therefore, $m_0(x_0) = 1$, as for any x_0 in $-b < x_0 < a$, eventual absorption at a or $-b$ must occur. When written out explicitly, the first terms of the series expansion Eq. (5.32) of u thus read

$$u(x_0) = 1 - s\, m_1(x_0) + \frac{1}{2}s^2\, m_2(x_0) - \ldots \qquad (5.33)$$

On the basis of Eq. (5.33), the expression $s\,u(x_0)$ on the left-hand side of Eq. (5.31) can be written as a power series in s starting with

$$s\,u(x_0) = s - s^2\,m_1(x_0) + \ldots \tag{5.34}$$

The major advantage of the representation of $u(x_0)$ in the last line of Eq. (5.32) is that terms involving s and x_0 appear separately. In particular, from the last line in Eq. (5.32), the first two derivatives of u with respect to x_0 are clearly given as

$$u'(x_0) = \sum_{i=0}^{\infty} \frac{(-s)^i}{i!}\,m_i'(x_0) \tag{5.35}$$

$$u''(x_0) = \sum_{i=0}^{\infty} \frac{(-s)^i}{i!}\,m_i''(x_0) \tag{5.36}$$

Specifically, remembering that the derivatives of $m_0(x_0) = 1$ vanish, the first terms of $u'(x_0)$ are given as

$$u'(x_0) = -s\,m_1'(x_0) + \frac{1}{2}s^2\,m_2'(x_0) - \ldots \tag{5.37}$$

and correspondingly we have

$$u''(x_0) = -s\,m_1''(x_0) + \frac{1}{2}s^2\,m_2''(x_0) - \ldots \tag{5.38}$$

Going back to Eq. (5.31), we can think of writing both the left-hand side and the right-hand side as a power series in s. The identity in Eq. (5.31) then means that the coefficients of each power s^i on both sides can be equated.

To see this operation more clearly, let us for the moment focus on the coefficients of the first power, s^1, on both sides of Eq. (5.31). From Eq. (5.34), we know that the coefficient of s^1 on the left-hand side of Eq. (5.31) is just 1. Similarly, from Eq. (5.38), we know that the coefficient of s^1 in $\frac{1}{2}\sigma^2(x_0)\,u''(x_0)$ is equal to $-\frac{1}{2}\sigma^2(x_0)\,m_1''(x_0)$. Finally, from Eq. (5.37), the coefficient of s^1 in $\mu(x_0)\,u'(x_0)$ equals $-\mu(x_0)\,m_1'(x_0)$. Equating these coefficients of s^1 on both sides of Eq. (5.31) and then multiplying by -1 give

$$\frac{1}{2}\sigma^2(x_0)\,m_1''(x_0) + \mu(x_0)\,m_1'(x_0) = -1 \tag{5.39}$$

Equation (5.39) is an ordinary first-order differential equation for $m_1'(x_0)$ which can, under wide regularity conditions, in principle be solved for any given functions $\sigma^2(x_0)$ and $\mu(x_0)$. This in turn means that we can also find the mean first-passage time $m_1(x_0)$ itself for any start point x_0 by integrating the solution $m_1'(x_0)$.

Equation (5.39) is essentially due to Darling and Siegert (1953) and represents one main approach to analyze diffusion process that are more general than the Wiener process. The derivation of Eq. (5.39) should make it clear that essentially the same approach can also be used to find higher moments of the first-passage time, by comparing the coefficients of higher powers s^i on both sides of Eq. (5.31). Note, however, that the corresponding equations for higher moments $m_i(x_0)$ are recursive, that is, to solve them, we need to know all lower moments $m_j(x_0)$ with $j < i$. For example, on comparing the coefficients of s^2 on both sides of Eq. (5.31), we get for the expected square $m_2(x_0)$ of the first-passage time

$$\sigma^2(x_0) \, m_2''(x_0) \; + \; \mu(x_0) \, m_2'(x_0) = -2m_1(x_0) \tag{5.40}$$

In order to solve Eq. (5.40) for $m_2(x_0)$, we first need to find $m_1(x_0)$ from Eq. (5.39).

In Chap. 6, we will study in some detail the appropriate boundary conditions for Eq. (5.39). There we will also see how the present approach can be adapted to handle absorption probabilities, conditional expectations, and reflecting barriers as well.

5.6 Exercises

1. Explain the analogies between x_0, k, and t in Eq. (5.17) (with $\mu = 0$) and the quantities r, m, and k in Eq. (2.57) for the discrete Ehrenfest model.
2. Explain why the OU process gets stuck at $x = 0$ when the restoring force k is a large, positive quantity.
3. Use a graphics tool to plot the (normal) distribution of $X(t)$ in the OU process for $x_0 = 100$, $\mu = 1.25$, $k = 0.125$, and $\sigma = 5$ at times $t = 1, 5, 10, 25, 50$. To which (normal) distribution does the process tend in the limit for large t?
4. Show that Eqs. (5.17) and (5.18) tend to $x_0 + \mu t$ and $\sigma^2 t$, respectively, when $k \to 0$.
5. Why does the variance of $X(t)$ in the OU process increase unboundedly with time when $k < 0$? What about $E[X(t)]$ in this case?
6. According to Eq. (5.17), the mean of $X(t)$ will not change across time when the start point (and thus constant mean) of the process is equal to μ/k. Explain the balance underlying the dynamics in this limiting case, and consider this behavior separately for positive and negative k.
7. Recover the results $E[X(\Delta t)] = x_0 + (\mu - kx_0)\Delta t$ and $\mathsf{Var}[X(\Delta t)] = \sigma^2 \Delta t$ by inserting into Eqs. (5.17) and (5.18) small values of Δt in place of t.
8. Compare Eq. (5.25) for the continuous Fisher–Wright model to its discrete counterpart Eq. (2.64) to explain the meaning of k in Eq. (5.19) in terms of the population size m of the discrete model.

9. In any individual realization, the Fisher–Wright process starting at x_0 will ultimately be fixated either in state $x = 0$ or in $x = 1$ and not change thereafter. Explain why then according to Eq. (5.25) the variance of $X(t)$ for large t is $x_0 (1 - x_0)$ and not zero?

10. Derive Eq. (5.40) from Eq. (5.31), using similar steps as those leading to Eq. (5.39), but focusing on the coefficients of s^2.

Chapter 6
Differential Equations for Probabilities and Means

6.1 Introduction

In Chap. 5, we have seen that diffusion processes with state-dependent drift or variance terms are characterized by the general forward and backward Equations (5.6) and (5.7), respectively. In many cases, their explicit solution under the appropriate initial and boundary conditions is difficult, complex, and will often require recourse to numerical techniques. One reaction to this situation is to avoid determining the full explicit transition or corresponding first-passage time density and instead to obtain information about absorption probabilities and mean first-passage times in a way that does not require the explicit solution, for example, of Eqs. (5.6) or (5.7). In this chapter, we will consider a practically important technique to this end that rests on a systematization and generalization of the basic approach described in Sect. 5.5.

In the following, we will consider diffusion processes $\{X(t), t \geq 0\}$ with infinitesimal drift $\mu(x)$ and infinitesimal variance $\sigma^2(x)$, starting at time $t = 0$ at position x_0 between two absorbing barriers placed at $-b < x_0 < a$. In the sequel, these barriers will not be explicitly varied, so that for simplicity, we will suppress in our notation a and b. As another notational simplification, we will in this chapter as well drop the index of x_0 and abbreviate simply as x the starting point $X(t = 0)$ of the process.

Let us denote as $g(t|x)$ the density of the first-passage time $\mathbf{T}$, that is, the time until the process first reaches one of the two barriers, no matter which. Clearly, this density will depend on the starting point x; therefore, the starting point will be explicitly represented in our notation. The event to absorb at the lower or upper barrier may be written more formally as $X(\mathbf{T}) = -b$ and $X(\mathbf{T}) = a$, respectively. For example, $X(\mathbf{T}) = a$ indicates that at the moment $\mathbf{T}$ when the first-passage took place, the position of the process was equal to a.

© Springer Nature Switzerland AG 2022
W. Schwarz, *Random Walk and Diffusion Models*,
https://doi.org/10.1007/978-3-031-12100-5_6

If a first passage occurs at time t, then the absorption happens either at the lower barrier $-b$ or at the upper barrier a, that is, $X(\mathbf{T}) = a$ or $X(\mathbf{T}) = -b$. Thus, let $g_+(t|x)$ be the density to absorb at time t at the upper barrier a. Similarly, let $g_-(t|x)$ be the density to absorb at time t at the lower barrier $-b$. Because absorbing at a and $-b$ are mutually exclusive events, we have

$$g(t|x) = g_-(t|x) + g_+(t|x) \tag{6.1}$$

Note that $g_-(t|x)$ and $g_+(t|x)$ do not integrate to unity across t. For example, $g_+(t|x)$ integrates to $\pi_+(x)$, the probability of absorbing (at some time) at a rather than at $-b$, when the start is at x. That is, $\pi_+(x)$ is the probability that $X(t)$ reaches the level a before it had ever reached the level $-b$. If we divide $g_+(t|x)$ by $\pi_+(x)$, then we get the regular conditional density (integrating to unity) of $\mathbf{T}$, given the absorption takes place at a. In contrast, because it is certain (probability of 1) that the process ultimately absorbs at the one or other barrier, the density $g(t|x)$ integrates to unity across t.

Extending the basic approach introduced and explained in Sect. 5.5, in the following, we will consider in detail the Laplace transforms u of these first-passage time densities. Specifically, let us denote as

$$u(x|s) = \int_0^\infty \exp(-st)\, g(t|x)\, dt$$

$$u_+(x|s) = \int_0^\infty \exp(-st)\, g_+(t|x)\, dt$$

$$u_-(x|s) = \int_0^\infty \exp(-st)\, g_-(t|x)\, dt \tag{6.2}$$

This somewhat elaborate notation underlines that u, u_+, and u_- depend not only on the starting state x but also on s.

Both $g(t|x)$ and also $g_-(t|x)$, $g_+(t|x)$ satisfy the backward partial differential equation (5.8) in the variables x (the start point, in the present notation) and t. We have seen in Sect. 5.5 that it follows from this fact that, for example, $u(x|s)$ satisfies the ordinary differential equation

$$\frac{1}{2}\sigma^2(x)u''(x|s) + \mu(x)u'(x|s) = s \cdot u(x|s) \tag{6.3}$$

and exactly corresponding equations hold for $u_-(x|s)$ and $u_+(x|s)$ as well. Note that in this equation, derivatives (indicated by primes) are taken with respect to the starting state x and that s plays the role of a fixed parameter. Specifically, Eq. (6.3) must hold for any $s \geq 0$ separately.

The functions u, u_-, and u_+ which appear in Eq. (6.3) contain implicitly important information about absorption probabilities and the distribution of the time at which absorption occurs. For example, note that for $s = 0$, we have

$$u_+(x|s = 0) = \int_0^\infty g_+(t|x)\, dt \qquad (6.4)$$

which is just the probability $\pi_+(x)$ to absorb (at any time) at the upper barrier a, considered as a function of the starting state x. In contrast to u_+, note from Eq. (6.2) that we must have $u(x|s = 0) = 1$ which trivially also satisfies Eq. (6.3).

Similarly, when we differentiate $u(x|s)$ with respect to s and evaluate the negative of this derivative at $s = 0$, we get from the definition of u in Eq. (6.2)

$$-\left. \frac{d}{ds} u(x|s) \right|_{s=0} = \int_0^\infty t\, g(t|x)\, dt \qquad (6.5)$$

which is evidently $m(x)$, the unconditional (i.e., irrespective of the barrier at which absorption takes place) mean first-passage time, $\mathsf{E}[\mathbf{T}]$, considered as a function of the start point x.

In contrast, the negative of the corresponding derivative of the function u_+ is equal to

$$m_+(x) = -\left. \frac{d}{ds} u_+(x|s) \right|_{s=0} = \int_0^\infty t\, g_+(t|x)\, dt \qquad (6.6)$$

As $g_+(t|x)$ integrates across t only to $\pi_+(x)$, not to unity, the expression $m_+(x)$ is equal to $\mathsf{E}[\mathbf{T}|X(\mathbf{T}) = a] \cdot \pi_+(x)$, that is, the conditional mean first-passage time given absorption at a, multiplied by the probability that the absorption takes place at this barrier. This may best be seen by rewriting the last expression in the equivalent form

$$m_+(x) = -\left. \frac{d}{ds} u_+(x|s) \right|_{s=0} = \int_0^\infty t\, \frac{g_+(t|x)}{\pi_+(x)}\, dt \cdot \pi_+(x) \qquad (6.7)$$

and noting that $g_+(t|x)/\pi_+(x)$ is the regular conditional density to absorb at time t, given the absorption takes places at a.

These considerations seem to suggest that to obtain useful information about absorption probabilities and first-passage times, it might be a viable approach to first derive the functions u, u_+, and u_- explicitly from Eq. (6.3) and then to determine their values, or the values of their s−derivative, specifically at $s = 0$. However, as we will illustrate in the next section, this seemingly most direct approach often leads to complex and unwieldy expressions, even in standard cases. This in turn will motivate us to look for more feasible and efficient routes, as suggested by the Darling and Siegert equations in Sect. 5.5.

6.2 Two Absorbing Barriers: Unconditional Results

In this section, we start from the ordinary differential equation (6.3) for the Laplace transform $u(x|s)$ of the first-passage time density $g(t|x)$ and show how we can actually determine u explicitly for the standard case of the Wiener process. To this end, we need to consider more generally—for any choice of $\mu(x)$ and $\sigma^2(x)$—the conditions that u must satisfy at the absorbing boundaries $-b$ and a; naturally, these conditions follow from the properties of $g(t|x)$ as the starting point x tends to $-b$ or a. Based on the properties of u discussed in the preceding Sect. 6.1, we will then derive information about the mean first-passage times from u.

6.2.1 Boundary Conditions and Explicit Solutions

As usual, an instructive special case to illustrate the basic approach is the Wiener process with drift, i.e., $\sigma^2(x) = \sigma^2$ and $\mu(x) = \mu$. To understand the general technique, let us consider Eq. (6.3) for u for this special case.

For the Wiener process, Eq. (6.3) takes the form

$$\frac{1}{2}\sigma^2 u''(x|s) + \mu u'(x|s) = s \cdot u(x|s) \tag{6.8}$$

For any fixed $s \geq 0$, this is an ordinary second-order differential equation for $u(x|s)$ in the variable x; its general solution is (cf., Stewart 2012, ch. 17)

$$u(x|s) = c_1 \cdot \exp(k_1 x) + c_2 \cdot \exp(k_2 x)$$
$$\text{where} \quad k_{1,2} = \frac{-\mu \pm \sqrt{\mu^2 + 2s\sigma^2}}{\sigma^2} \tag{6.9}$$

To determine the two constants c_1 and c_2, we need to consider the nature of $u(x|s)$ at the absorbing boundaries at $-b$ and a. When $X(t)$ starts either at $-b$ or at a, the process will be absorbed immediately. In these cases, as x tends to $-b$ or to a, the function g will tend to a density still covering the area 1, but being arbitrarily narrowly confined to an interval concentrated at the origin. This limit is called a $\delta(t)$−function with a unit impulse at $t = 0$, and we may think of it as a rectangle at the origin of decreasing width and increasing height so that its area remains 1. From this conceptualization, it may be seen (cf., Exercise 10) that the Laplace transform u of a $\delta(t)$−function is unity. Thus, the boundary conditions for u at $x = -b$ and at $x = a$ are

$$u(-b|s) = 1 \quad \text{and} \quad u(a|s) = 1 \tag{6.10}$$

and we can use these two boundary conditions to determine c_1 and c_2 in Eq. (6.9). In the case of general $\mu(x)$ and $\sigma^2(x)$, Eq. (6.3) is more complex, but the basic reasoning regarding the nature of $g(t|x)$, and thus of $u(x|s)$, in the limit of $x \to -b$ and $x \to a$ remains exactly the same. In particular, the boundary conditions for $u(x|s)$ at the absorbing barriers $x = a$ and $x = -b$ will still be given by Eq. (6.10).

Inserting the boundary conditions into the general solution Eq. (6.9) for $u(x|s)$ with $x = -b$ and $x = a$, we get two equations in the two unknowns c_1 and c_2. From the spatial homogeneity of the Wiener process (i.e., σ^2 and μ do not vary with x), we can without loss of generality set $b = 0$ and for this case get the solution

$$c_1 = \frac{1 - \exp(k_2 a)}{\exp(k_1 a) - \exp(k_2 a)} \quad \text{and} \quad c_2 = 1 - c_1$$

Having fully determined $u(x|s)$, we could now in principle find from the derivatives of u with respect to s properties of the first-passage time $\mathbf{T}$, such as its unconditional mean. Note, however, that these derivatives involve $k_{1,2}$, which in turn are functions of s (cf., Eq. (6.9)). It is this complex dependence on s that renders the approach via the full determination and subsequent analysis of u rather tedious, even in the standard case of the Wiener process, and much more so for the case of general $\mu(x)$ and $\sigma^2(x)$. Therefore, we next turn to the general approach exemplified by the Darling and Siegert equations in Sect. 5.5.

6.2.2 Mean Unconditional First-Passage Time

In Sect. 5.5, we have seen that from the differential Eq. (6.3) for the Laplace transform $u(x|s)$, we can derive the general first-order Equation (5.39) for $m(x)$, the mean first-passage time $\mathbf{T}$, and in fact recursive equations for higher moments as well, such as Eq. (5.40) for $E[\mathbf{T}^2]$.

In the following, we will focus on the mean first-passage time, $m(x)$. According to Eq. (5.39), we have

$$\frac{1}{2}\sigma^2(x) \cdot m''(x) + \mu(x) \cdot m'(x) = -1 \tag{6.11}$$

Equation (6.11) is a basic result for mean first-passage times in diffusion processes. Formally, given $\sigma^2(x)$ and $\mu(x)$, it is an ordinary first-order differential equation for $m'(x)$. Therefore, Eq. (6.11) can routinely be solved for $m'(x)$; integrating the solution once more gives $m(x)$.

Solving Eq. (6.11) in the way suggested produces two integration constants. To determine them, we need to consider the boundary values of $m(x)$ at the absorbing barriers. As the process $X(t)$ will be immediately absorbed when it starts at $-b$ or at a, the appropriate boundary conditions for $m(x)$ at $x = -b$ and $x = a$ are clearly

$$m(-b) = 0 \quad \text{and} \quad m(a) = 0 \tag{6.12}$$

Of course, depending on $\sigma^2(x)$ and $\mu(x)$, explicit solutions to Eq. (6.11) may become unwieldy, and in these cases, numerical routines to solve this equation or to compute its formal solution can be preferable. A few examples will serve to illustrate typical ways in which Eq. (6.11) is applied.

6.2.3   Examples

For the case of the Wiener process, we have $\mu(x) = \mu, \sigma^2(x) = \sigma^2$. Choosing $b = 0$ for the lower barrier, the solution of Eq. (6.11) satisfying the boundary conditions $m(0) = m(a) = 0$ is

$$m(x) = \frac{a}{\mu} \left[\frac{1 - \exp\left(-\frac{2\mu x}{\sigma^2}\right)}{1 - \exp\left(-\frac{2\mu a}{\sigma^2}\right)} - \frac{x}{a} \right] \tag{6.13}$$

which may be shown to correspond to Eq. (4.50). The typical inverted-u shape of the function $m(x)$ is shown in Fig. 6.1.

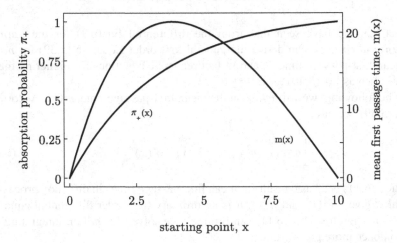

Fig. 6.1 Mean first-passage time (right ordinate) and absorption probability (left ordinate) for the Wiener process, $\mu(x) = \mu = 0.15$, $\sigma^2(x) = \sigma^2 = 1$. The peaked curve shows the mean first-passage time $m(x) = \mathsf{E}[T|X(0) = x]$ as a function of the start position x (abscissa) of the Wiener process between the absorbing barriers at $b = 0$ and $a = 10$ (cf., Eq. (6.13)). The increasing curve shows the probability $\pi_+(x)$ to absorb at the upper barrier a (cf., Eq. (6.26))

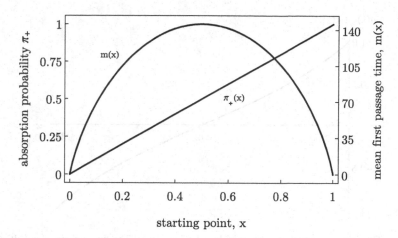

starting point, x

Fig. 6.2 Mean first-passage time (right ordinate) and absorption probability (left ordinate) for the Fisher–Wright model, $\mu(x) = 0$, $\sigma^2(x) = kx(1-x)$, with $k = 1/100$. The peaked curve shows the mean first-passage time $m(x) = E[T|X(0) = x]$ as a function of the start position x (abscissa) of the process between the absorbing barriers at $b = 0$ and $a = 1$ (cf., Eq. (6.15)). The linear curve shows the probability $\pi_+(x)$ to absorb at the upper barrier $a = 1$ (cf., Eq. (6.25))

As a second example, consider the Fisher–Wright model of random genetic drift as discussed in Sects. 2.5.2 and 5.3.2. In the present notation, this model considers the diffusion process characterized by $\mu(x) = 0$ and $\sigma^2(x) = kx(1-x)$ between the barriers $b = 0$ and $a = 1$. For this model, Eq. (6.11) for $m(x)$ simplifies to

$$m''(x) = -\frac{2}{kx(1-x)} \tag{6.14}$$

with $m(0) = m(1) = 0$. Its solution

$$m(x) = -\frac{2}{k} \left[x \ln(x) + (1-x) \ln(1-x) \right] \tag{6.15}$$

is shown in Fig. 6.2, revealing that the mean first-passage time decreases symmetrically as the starting point x moves away from the midpoint $\frac{1}{2}$.

As a final example, consider the case of a diffusion process characterized by $\mu(x) = \cot(x)$ and $\sigma^2 = 1$ between two absorbing barriers at $-b = \pi/4$ and $a = 3\pi/4$. These assumptions model a simple built-in regression (mean-reverting) effect toward $x = \pi/2$. As shown in Fig. 6.3, $\mu(x)$ is positive below $\pi/2$ and negative above $\pi/2$, thus driving in both cases the process toward $\pi/2$.

For this model, the corresponding Eq. (6.11) for $m(x)$ becomes

$$\frac{1}{2} \cdot m_1''(x) + \cot(x) \cdot m_1'(x) = -1 \tag{6.16}$$

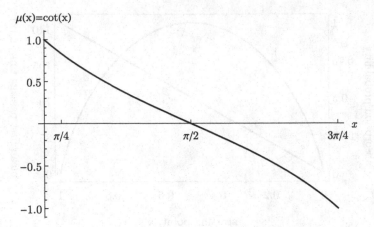

Fig. 6.3 The diffusion model characterized by $\mu(x) = \cot(x)$. The figure shows the drift $\mu(x)$ (ordinate) as a function of the spatial position x (abscissa) between the absorbing barriers at $-b = \frac{\pi}{4}$ and $a = \frac{3\pi}{4}$. Note that $\mu(x)$ is positive to the left of $\pi/2$ and negative to the right of $\pi/2$, thus driving in both cases the process toward $\pi/2$

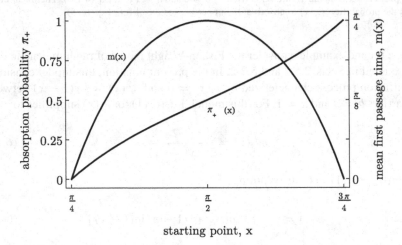

Fig. 6.4 Mean first-passage time (right ordinate) and absorption probability (left ordinate) for the diffusion model $\mu(x) = \cot(x)$, $\sigma^2(x) = 1$. The peaked curve shows the mean first-passage time $m(x) = E[T|X(0) = x]$ as a function of the start position x (abscissa) of the process between the absorbing barriers at $-b = \pi/4$ and $a = 3\pi/4$ (cf., Eq. (6.17)). The increasing curve shows the probability $\pi_+(x)$ to absorb at the upper barrier a (cf., Eq. (6.27))

with $m(\pi/4) = m(3\pi/4) = 0$. The solution

$$m(x) = \frac{\pi}{4} + \left(x - \frac{\pi}{2}\right)\cot(x) \tag{6.17}$$

is shown in Fig. 6.4, indicating a similarly symmetrical dependence of the mean first-passage time on the starting point x as in the previous example.

A conspicuous feature of these examples is the similar shape of $m(x)$ in all three cases, despite the rather different assumptions about $\mu(x)$ and $\sigma^2(x)$. In all three cases, $m(x)$ increases from $m(-b) = 0$ toward a unique maximum at x_m and then decreases to $m(a) = 0$. This feature is not accidental. The basic differential Eq. (6.11) for $m(x)$ implies that at any extremal point x_m such that $m'(x_m) = 0$, it must be the case that $m''(x_m) = -2/\sigma^2(x_m) < 0$ which means that any such extremal point is a maximum. As two maxima of a continuous function necessarily enclose a minimum in between, this means that $m(x)$ has only one maximum. Of course, different diffusion models can still differ vastly with respect to other features, such as the location, x_m, or the height, $m(x_m)$, of the maximum.

6.3 Two Absorbing Barriers: Conditional Results

The results in Sect. 6.2.2 refer to unconditional mean first-passage times, ignoring the barrier at which $X(t)$ absorbs. In many contexts, we would like to know how long it takes on average to absorption in all those cases in which this absorption took place, say, at the upper barrier a. In the notation used above, the associated conditional expectation may thus be expressed as $E[T|X(T) = a]$. An important step to compute it is to first find the probability $P[X(T) = a]$ of the event on which this expectation is conditioned, that is, absorption at barrier a. As before, to indicate the dependence on the starting state $X(0) = x$, we will use $\pi_+(x)$ to denote this probability.

To obtain absorption probabilities and conditional mean first-passage times, we need to consider the Laplace transforms of the densities $g_+(t|x)$ and $g_-(t|x)$, that is, $u_+(x|s)$ and $u_-(x|s)$. Similar to $g(t|x)$, the functions $g_+(t|x)$ and $g_-(t|x)$ satisfy the backward equation (5.8) in the variables x and t. This implies that just as Eq. (6.3) holds for $u(x|s)$, the functions $u_+(x|s)$ and $u_-(x|s)$ also satisfy the ordinary differential equations

$$\frac{1}{2}\sigma^2(x)u_+''(x|s) + \mu(x)u_+'(x|s) = s \cdot u_+(x|s) \tag{6.18}$$

$$\frac{1}{2}\sigma^2(x)u_-''(x|s) + \mu(x)u_-'(x|s) = s \cdot u_-(x|s) \tag{6.19}$$

in the start variable x for any $s \geq 0$. In the following, we will illustrate the main points for u_+, but it is understood that analogous considerations apply to u_- as well.

6.3.1 Boundary Conditions and Solutions

As in the case of $u(x|s)$, we need to consider the behavior of $u_+(x|s)$ at the absorbing boundaries at $-b$ and a. If $X(t)$ starts at $x = -b$, it will never absorb at barrier a, and so the density $g_+(t|x) = 0$; in view of Eq. (6.2), this implies that $u_+(-b|s) = 0$. On the other hand, if $X(t)$ starts at a, the process will be absorbed immediately; as explained in the reasoning leading to Eq. (6.10), the Laplace transform u_+ of g_+ is then unity. In sum, the boundary conditions for u_+ are

$$u_+(-b|s) = 0 \quad \text{and} \quad u_+(a|s) = 1 \qquad (6.20)$$

For u_-, the reasoning is exactly reversed, leading to the boundary conditions

$$u_-(-b|s) = 1 \quad \text{and} \quad u_-(a|s) = 0 \qquad (6.21)$$

Note that just as the densities g_- and g_+ add up to g (see Eq. (6.1)) so their Laplace transforms u_- and u_+ add up to give u. This means that, in particular, the boundary conditions for u_- and u_+ both at $x = -b$ and at $x = a$ add up to give those of u.

6.3.2 Absorption Probabilities

We noticed in Eq. (6.4) that for $s = 0$, the function u_+ reduces to the integral across $g_+(t|x)$ with respect to t. Thus, $u_+(x|0)$ represents the absorption probability $\pi_+(x)$, to reach the barrier a before having reached $-b$. Now, Eq. (6.18) holds for any $s \geq 0$; setting, specifically, $s = 0$, we get

$$\frac{1}{2}\sigma^2(x)\pi_+''(x) + \mu(x)\pi_+'(x) = 0 \qquad (6.22)$$

This is a homogeneous first-order differential equation that can always be solved for $\pi_+'(x)$. The solution is seen to be

$$\pi_+'(x) = C \exp\left[-2\int^x \frac{\mu(u)}{\sigma^2(u)}\,du\right] \qquad (6.23)$$

Integrating this solution formally, and applying the two boundary conditions from Eq. (6.20) for $u_+(x|0) = \pi_+(x)$, the general solution for the absorption probability satisfying $\pi_+(-b) = 0$ and $\pi_+(a) = 1$ is

$$\pi_+(x) = \frac{L(x)}{L(a)}, \quad \text{where} \quad L(x) = \int_{-b}^{x} \exp\left[-2\int_{-b}^{v} \frac{\mu(u)}{\sigma^2(u)}\,du\right]dv \qquad (6.24)$$

In Eq. (6.24), the denominator $L(a)$ is positive, and so $\pi_+(x)$ increases if $L(x)$ increases. Now, from Eq. (6.24), we see that $L'(x)$ is clearly positive. Thus, $\pi_+(x)$ generally increases in x, as we would expect: the closer to a the process starts, the more likely it is that it absorbs at this barrier.

The following elementary probabilistic argument supports this conclusion. Consider two points x and $y > x$ in $[-b, a]$. Starting from x, any path ultimately absorbing at a must necessarily first reach y without previously reaching the absorbing barrier at $-b$. According to Eq. (6.24), this event clearly has probability $L(x)/L(y) < 1$. Continuing from y on, the path must then reach a before reaching $-b$ which in turn has probability $L(y)/L(a)$, the product giving the required overall probability $\pi_+(x) = L(x)/L(a)$. This means that $L(x)/L(a) < L(y)/L(a)$, that is, $\pi_+(x) < \pi_+(y)$, as is clear from the fact that $L'(x) > 0$.

A few examples serve to illustrate the result Eq. (6.24). For a drift-free process, $\mu(x) = 0$, the solution (for any $\sigma^2(x) > 0$) is clearly given by

$$\pi_+(x) = \frac{x+b}{a+b} \tag{6.25}$$

One example of this case is the Fisher–Wright model shown in Fig. 6.2, for which $b = 0$ and $a = 1$, and so $\pi_+(x) = x$.

For the Wiener process with drift, we have $\mu(x) = \mu, \sigma^2(x) = \sigma^2$. Choosing $b = 0$ for the lower barrier, we find $L(x) = 1 - \exp\left(-\frac{2\mu x}{\sigma^2}\right)$, and so the absorption probability is seen to be

$$\pi_+(x) = \frac{1 - \exp\left(-\frac{2\mu x}{\sigma^2}\right)}{1 - \exp\left(-\frac{2\mu a}{\sigma^2}\right)} \tag{6.26}$$

The typical form of Eq. (6.26) is illustrated in Fig. 6.1. The result conforms to Eq. (4.44) when we adjust the barriers to the present notation, $a' = a - x$ and $b' = x$. As $\mu \to 0$, this expression tends to $\pi_+(x) = \frac{x}{a}$, consistent with the solution Eq. (6.25) that is obtained from Eq. (6.24) by setting $\mu(x) = 0$.

For the simple regression-to-the mean model, characterized by $\mu(x) = \cot(x)$, $\sigma^2 = 1$, and absorbing barriers placed at $-b = \pi/4$ and $a = 3\pi/4$, we find

$$\pi_+(x) = \frac{1}{2}\left[1 - \cot(x)\right] \tag{6.27}$$

The characteristic form of Eq. (6.27) with its steeper ends and flatter middle portion is shown in Fig. 6.4.

6.3.3 Mean Conditional First-Passage Time

To derive mean conditional first-passage times, the procedure is similar in principle to the one in Sect. 6.2.2, but it differs in some characteristic features which we next discuss in more detail. To be more specific, we again first focus on the absorption at the upper barrier a and thus on the associated Laplace transform $u_+(x|s)$.

We concluded above from Eq. (6.4) that for $s = 0$, the function $u_+(x|s)$ reduces to $\pi_+(x)$. Also, Eq. (6.7) indicated that $g_+(t|x)/\pi_+(x)$ is the regular (integrating to unity) conditional density of the first-passage time, given that absorption occurs at a. This means that, for example, the quantity $m_+(x) = \int_0^\infty t\, g_+(t|x)dt$ does not itself represent the mean conditional first-passage time; rather, it represents $E[\mathbf{T}|X(\mathbf{T}) = a] \cdot \pi_+(x)$. However, from $m_+(x)$, it is then easy to find the conditional expectation $E[\mathbf{T}|X(\mathbf{T}) = a]$ itself, at least after $\pi_+(x)$ has been determined from Eq. (6.24).

We next use these background results to modify appropriately the basic approach that was explained in Sect. 5.5 to find the unconditional moments of the first-passage time. That is, our main strategy is again to write $u_+(x|s)$ as a power series in s, with coefficients which depend on the starting point x. As for any regular power series, for $s = 0$, it must reduce to the coefficient of s^0, which from Eq. (6.4) is equal to $u_+(x|0) = \pi_+(x)$. Similarly, the first derivative of this power series, again evaluated at $s = 0$, must reduce to the coefficient of s^1, which from Eq. (6.6) we know is equal to $-m_+(x)$. We may thus write the initial terms of the power series for $u_+(x|s)$ in the form

$$u_+(x|s) = \pi_+(x) \cdot s^0 - m_+(x) \cdot s^1 + \ldots \tag{6.28}$$

Inserting next this series representation into the basic differential equation (6.18) for $u_+(s|x)$

$$\frac{1}{2}\sigma^2(x)u_+''(x|s) + \mu(x)u_+'(x|s) = s \cdot u_+(x|s)$$

we get

$$\frac{1}{2}\sigma^2(x) \cdot \left[\pi_+''(x) \cdot s^0 - m_+''(x) \cdot s^1 + \ldots\right] + \mu(x) \cdot \left[\pi_+'(x) \cdot s^0 - m_+'(x) \cdot s^1 + \ldots\right]$$

$$= s^1 \cdot \pi_+(x) - \ldots \tag{6.29}$$

On comparing the coefficients for s^0 on both sides, we recover Eq. (6.22)

$$\frac{1}{2}\sigma^2(x) \cdot \pi_+''(x) + \mu(x) \cdot \pi_+'(x) = 0$$

for the absorption probabilities $\pi_+(x)$.

Next, comparing the coefficients of s^1 on both sides of Eq. (6.29), we find

$$\frac{1}{2}\sigma^2(x) \cdot m_+''(x) + \mu(x) \cdot m_+'(x) = -\pi_+(x) \tag{6.30}$$

Equation (6.30) represents the "conditional" counterpart to Eq. (6.11) for the unconditional mean first-passage time, $m(x)$. Like Eq. (6.11), it is an ordinary first-order differential equation for $m'_+(x)$ that can in principle routinely be solved, after we have first determined $\pi_+(x)$ from Eq. (6.24). However, the dependence of the right-hand side on x makes Eq. (6.30) more complex than the corresponding Eq. (6.11) for unconditional means. This will be especially true if the solution for $\pi_+(x)$ obtained from Eq. (6.24) is itself already an unwieldy expression.

6.3.4 Boundary Conditions for the Conditional Case

Next, we consider the appropriate boundary conditions that we need in order to solve Eq. (6.30) for $m_+(x)$. As $X(t)$ is immediately absorbed when it starts at a, the conditional expectation $\mathsf{E}[\mathbf{T}|X(\mathbf{T}) = a] = 0$. For the same reason, we clearly have $\pi_+(a) = 1$. According to Eq. (6.7), we have

$$m_+(x) = \mathsf{E}[\mathbf{T}|X(\mathbf{T}) = a] \cdot \pi_+(x) \tag{6.31}$$

and looking specifically at this equation for $x = a$, we find the boundary condition $m_+(a) = 0 \cdot 1 = 0$.

The boundary behavior of $m_+(x)$ at $x = -b$ follows from similar reasoning. Whenever $X(t)$ starts in the immediate neighborhood of $-b$, the conditional expectation $\mathsf{E}[\mathbf{T}|X(\mathbf{T}) = a]$ will clearly take some finite positive value. At the same time, $\pi_+(x)$ evidently tends to zero as x tends to $-b$. Therefore, the product on the right-hand side of Eq. (6.31) will tend to $m_+(-b) = 0$. Another way of understanding this boundary condition is to note that if $X(t)$ starts right at $-b$, then the density $g_+(t|-b) = 0$ for all t because the process will then never absorb at a. From the defining Eq. (6.2), we see that this implies that $u_+(-b|s) = 0$, too. This in turn means that in the power series development of $u_+(-b|s)$, the coefficient of s^1 must be equal to zero; by Eq. (6.28), this coefficient is equal to $-m_+(-b)$. In summary then we get for $m_+(x)$ the boundary conditions

$$m_+(-b) = 0 \quad \text{and} \quad m_+(a) = 0 \tag{6.32}$$

Note, however, that, in particular, the boundary condition at $x = -b$ does *not* mean that the corresponding conditional expectation $\mathsf{E}[\mathbf{T}|X(\mathbf{T}) = a]$ itself equals zero. In fact, Eq. (6.31) indicates that $\mathsf{E}[\mathbf{T}|X(\mathbf{T}) = a]$ is determined as the limit $x \to -b$ of $m_+(x)/\pi_+(x)$, an expression in which numerator and denominator individually tend to zero.

We again consider a few examples to illustrate the way in which Eqs. (6.30) and (6.32) are used to obtain the conditional expectation $\mathsf{E}[\mathbf{T}|X(\mathbf{T}) = a]$.

6.3.5   Examples

For the Wiener process with drift, we have $\mu(x) = \mu$ and $\sigma^2(x) = \sigma^2$. Choosing $b = 0$ for the lower barrier, we had determined $\pi_+(x)$ in Eq. (6.26). Therefore, Eq. (6.30) takes the form of

$$\frac{1}{2}\sigma^2 \cdot m_+''(x) + \mu \cdot m_+'(x) = -\frac{1 - \exp\left(-\frac{2\mu x}{\sigma^2}\right)}{1 - \exp\left(-\frac{2\mu a}{\sigma^2}\right)} \tag{6.33}$$

The solution of this equation which satisfies Eq. (6.32) is

$$m_+(x) = \frac{1 - \exp\left(-\frac{2\mu x}{\sigma^2}\right)}{1 - \exp\left(-\frac{2\mu a}{\sigma^2}\right)} \frac{1}{\mu} \left[a \coth\left(\frac{\mu a}{\sigma^2}\right) - x \coth\left(\frac{\mu x}{\sigma^2}\right) \right] \tag{6.34}$$

According to Eq. (6.31), to find the conditional expectation, we need to divide $m_+(x)$ by $\pi_+(x)$ and get

$$\mathsf{E}[T|X(T) = a] = \frac{1}{\mu} \left[a \coth\left(\frac{\mu a}{\sigma^2}\right) - x \coth\left(\frac{\mu x}{\sigma^2}\right) \right] \tag{6.35}$$

Figure 6.5 shows a typical example of Eq. (6.35). To further simplify this solution, we define the auxiliary function $g(z) = z \coth\left(\frac{\mu z}{\sigma^2}\right)$. We may then write the mean conditional first-passage time more compactly as

$$\mathsf{E}[T|X(T) = a] = \frac{1}{\mu} \cdot [g(a) - g(x)] \tag{6.36}$$

It is easy to verify that Eq. (6.35) corresponds to the earlier result Eq. (4.46) with $a' = a - x$ and $b' = x$ (cf., Eqs. (4.48 and 4.49)). Using the form of Eq. (6.36), it is particularly easy to derive the limit $\mu \to 0$, equal to

$$\lim_{\mu \to 0} \mathsf{E}[T|X(T) = a] = \frac{a^2 - x^2}{3\sigma^2} \tag{6.37}$$

Of course, the same result is obtained when the differential Eq. (6.30) for $m_+(x)$ is solved with $\sigma^2(x) = \sigma^2$ and $\mu(x) = 0$ under the boundary conditions indicated in Eq. (6.32), and then divided by $\pi_+(x) = \frac{x}{a}$.

An instructive feature of this example is as follows. First note that from Eq. (6.26), we have $\pi_+(x) \to 0$ as $x \to 0$, as expected. In spite of this zero limit, it is still true that the conditional mean $m_+(x)/\pi_+(x)$ in Eq. (6.35) tends to a finite limit as $x \to 0$, namely, to $(1/\mu^2)[(\mu a) \coth(\mu a/\sigma^2) - \sigma^2]$. For example, as $\mu \to 0$, this finite limit will be $\frac{a^2}{3\sigma^2}$, as is obvious from Eq. (6.37). If $X(t)$ starts at some x close

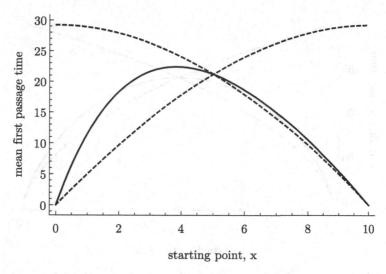

Fig. 6.5 Conditional mean first-passage time (ordinate) as a function of the starting position x (abscissa) for the Wiener process, $\mu(x) = \mu = 0.15$, $\sigma^2(x) = \sigma^2 = 1$, with absorbing barriers placed at $b = 0$ and $a = 10$. The declining broken line shows the conditional mean first-passage time given that the absorption occurs at $a = 10$ (cf., Eq. (6.35)). The increasing broken line shows the conditional mean first-passage time given that the absorption occurs at $b = 0$. The peaked full line refers to the unconditional mean first-passage time, equal to the weighted (by $\pi_+(x)$ and $1 - \pi_+(x)$) average of the two conditional means. The conditional curves necessarily intersect at the same point where both in turn intersect the curve for the unconditional mean

to $b = 0$, we would still expect the (conditional) expectation of the first-passage time to be finite in those rare cases in which the process ultimately absorbs at a, even if the probability $\pi_+(x)$ of this event is very small.

For the Fisher–Wright model, we have $\mu(x) = 0$, $\sigma^2(x) = kx(1 - x)$, with absorbing barriers placed at $b = 0$ and $a = 1$. We know from Eq. (6.25) that for this model, $\pi_+(x) = x$, and so Eq. (6.30) now takes the form

$$\frac{1}{2}kx(1 - x) \cdot m''_+(x) = -x \tag{6.38}$$

with $m_+(0) = m_+(1) = 0$. The solution is

$$m_+(x) = -\frac{2}{k}(1 - x)\ln(1 - x) \tag{6.39}$$

From Eq. (6.31), the conditional expectation of the time to reach the barrier at $a = 1$ is again obtained by dividing $m_+(x)$ by $\pi_+(x) = x$, giving

$$\mathsf{E}[\mathbf{T}|X(\mathbf{T}) = a] = -\frac{2}{k}\frac{1 - x}{x}\ln(1 - x) \tag{6.40}$$

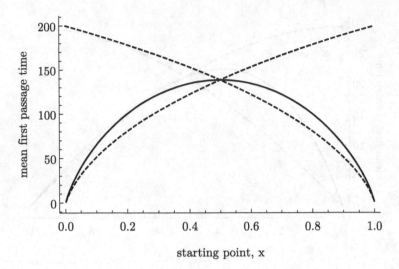

Fig. 6.6 Conditional mean first-passage time (ordinate) as a function of the starting position x (abscissa) for the Fisher–Wright model, $\mu(x) = 0$, $\sigma^2(x) = kx(1-x)$, with $k = 1/100$; the absorbing barriers are placed at $b = 0$ and $a = 1$. The declining broken line shows the conditional mean first-passage time given that the absorption occurs at $a = 1$ (cf., Eq. (6.40)). The increasing broken line shows the conditional mean first-passage time given that the absorption occurs at $b = 0$. The peaked full line refers to the unconditional mean first-passage time, equal to the weighted (by $\pi_+(x)$ and $1 - \pi_+(x)$) average of the two conditional means

This function is shown in Fig. 6.6. Note again that although $m_+(x)$ and $\pi_+(x)$ individually both tend to zero as $x \to 0$, their ratio $\mathsf{E}[\mathbf{T}|X(\mathbf{T}) = 1]$ tends to $2/k$.

For the regression-type model characterized by $\mu(x) = \cot(x)$, $\sigma^2 = 1$, the absorbing barriers are placed at $-b = \pi/4$ and $a = 3\pi/4$. For this model, $\pi_+(x)$ is given by Eq. (6.27), and the basic Eq. (6.30) then reads

$$\frac{1}{2} \cdot m_+''(x) + \cot(x) \cdot m_+'(x) = -\frac{1}{2}[1 - \cot(x)] \tag{6.41}$$

The solution of this equation satisfying the boundary conditions Eq. (6.32) is

$$m_+(x) = \frac{1}{2}[1 + \cot(x)] \cdot \left(x - \frac{\pi}{4}\right) \tag{6.42}$$

From Eq. (6.27) for $\pi_+(x)$, we then obtain via Eq. (6.31)

$$\mathsf{E}[\mathbf{T}|X(\mathbf{T}) = a] = \frac{1 + \cot(x)}{1 - \cot(x)} \cdot \left(x - \frac{\pi}{4}\right) \tag{6.43}$$

In Fig. 6.7, the conditional expectation $\mathsf{E}[\mathbf{T}|X(\mathbf{T}) = a]$ is shown as a function of the starting state $X(0) = x$.

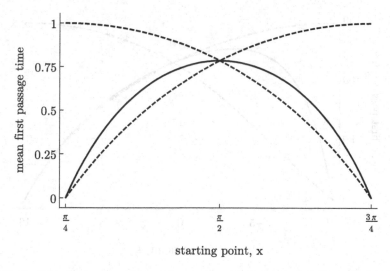

Fig. 6.7 Conditional mean first-passage time (ordinate) as a function of the starting position x (abscissa) for the diffusion model $\mu(x) = \cot(x)$, $\sigma^2(x) = 1$; the absorbing barriers are placed at $-b = \pi/4$ and $a = 3\pi/4$. The declining broken line shows the conditional mean first-passage time given that the absorption occurs at a (cf., Eq. (6.43)). The increasing broken line shows the conditional mean first-passage time given that the absorption occurs at $-b$. The peaked full line refers to the unconditional mean first-passage time, equal to the weighted (by $\pi_+(x)$ and $1-\pi_+(x)$) average of the two conditional means

A conspicuous feature apparent in Figs. 6.5, 6.6, and 6.7 is the symmetry of the conditional means, given absorption at a vs. $-b$, and the implied fact that these curves meet at the midpoint $(a - b)/2$ in between the two barriers. This is indeed a symmetry property that holds exactly, for example, for the Wiener process. However, as is illustrated in Fig. 6.8, for other diffusion models such as the OU process described in Sect. 5.3.1, this property does not hold.

6.4   One Absorbing and One Reflecting Barrier

In many modeling contexts involving an absorbing barrier, it is unrealistic to assume that the state variable of the diffusion process under study can move to any distance away from that barrier. Many naturally occurring states defined, for example, by weight, energy, size, or number are by definition restricted to be positive or are limited from below (or above) in other ways. As we discussed in Sects. 4.3 and 4.5–4.6, in these situations, a more realistic model may incorporate a *reflecting* barrier. To be specific, in the following, we will assume that the upper barrier a is absorbing and that $-b$ is reflecting.

Under this scenario, elementary considerations show that under minimal regularity conditions, it is certain that the process will ultimately absorb at a. A

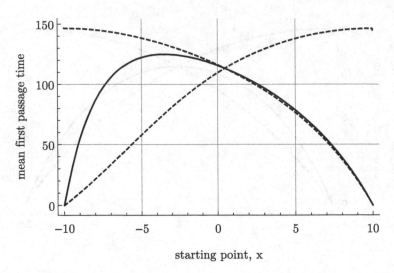

Fig. 6.8 Conditional mean first-passage time (ordinate) as a function of the starting position x (abscissa) for the OU process with $\mu(x) = 0.1 - 0.015x$, $\sigma^2(x) = 1$; the absorbing barriers are placed at $-b = -10$ and $a = 10$. The declining broken line shows the conditional mean first-passage time given that the absorption occurs at a. The increasing broken line shows the conditional mean first-passage time given that the absorption occurs at $-b$. The peaked full line refers to the unconditional mean first-passage time, equal to the weighted (by $\pi_+(x)$ and $1 - \pi_+(x)$) average of the two conditional means. The conditional curves necessarily intersect at the same point where both in turn intersect the curve for the unconditional mean, but for the OU model, this point is not half-way between the two absorbing barriers

main conceptual implication then is that the conditional mean first-passage time necessarily coincides with the unconditional mean first-passage time. The nature of the barriers delimiting the state space of the process does not affect the local dynamics governing $X(t)$ away from the boundaries. Thus, the first-passage time density $g_+(t|x)$ to the barrier at a still satisfies the basic backward Eq. (5.8), and so its Laplace transform $u_+(x|s)$ satisfies Eq. (6.18). Setting $s = 0$ in Eq. (6.18), this means that formally the differential Eq. (6.22) for $\pi_+(x)$ remains valid

$$\frac{1}{2}\sigma^2(x)\,\pi_+''(x) \,+\, \mu(x)\,\pi_+'(x) = 0 \qquad (6.44)$$

The fact that there is only a single absorbing barrier at which for any starting point x the process will ultimately absorb may be expressed more formally by $\pi_+(x) = 1$. Conceptually, this implies that the density $g_+(t|x)$ of the first-passage time to the absorbing barrier a is regular, that is, it integrates to 1. Note that trivially $\pi_+(x) = 1$ satisfies Eq. (6.44).

Next, we note that for $\pi_+(x) = 1$, Eq. (6.30) for conditional mean first-passage times simplifies to Eq. (6.11) for unconditional mean first-passage times. Thus, in the presence of a reflecting barrier at $-b$, the basic differential equation governing the mean first-passage time $m(x)$ to the barrier a is the same as for unconditional mean first-passage times with two absorbing barriers, namely,

$$\frac{1}{2}\sigma^2(x)\,m''(x) + \mu(x)\,m'(x) = -1 \tag{6.45}$$

What, however, differs from the case of the unconditional mean first-passage time between two absorbing barriers are the boundary conditions under which we now have to solve (6.45). To address this point, we next consider what are the appropriate boundary conditions for Eq. (6.45) if the lower barrier at $-b$ is reflecting.

6.4.1 Boundary Conditions and Solutions

The boundary condition at $x = a$ is evidently $m(a) = 0$, namely, when the diffusion process $X(t)$ starts right at the absorbing barrier at a. In contrast, the boundary condition at $x = -b$ is not evident. To understand its nature, it is helpful to reconsider the basic dynamics of the process near $-b$ and the meaning of a reflecting barrier. Ultimately, this consideration will show that the required boundary condition is $m'(-b) = 0$.

As we are interested in the behavior of $m(x)$ close to $-b$, let us assume that at time $t = 0$, the process starts at the reflecting barrier, that is, $X(0) = -b$. Thus, the local infinitesimal drift is $\mu(-b)$, and the infinitesimal variance is $\sigma^2(-b)$. We reason heuristically and consider the discrete approximation in which in any small time interval Δt, a step of size Δx is made that with probability $p(\Delta t)$ is to the right and with probability $1 - p(\Delta t)$ to the left. As we have seen in Sect. 4.1.1, a meaningful finite limit for small Δt requires that Δx is of the order of $\sqrt{\Delta t}$ and also that the step probability $p(\Delta t) \to \frac{1}{2}$ as $\Delta t \to 0$.

Now, because the lower barrier is reflecting, during the interval $[0, \Delta t]$, the process will with probability $1 - p(\Delta t)$ bump into the reflecting barrier and thus remain at $-b$, and with probability $p(\Delta t)$, it moves upward to reach the position $-b + \Delta x$. In the first case, the overall mean first-passage time to a will be equal to $\Delta t + m(-b)$, and in the second case, it is $\Delta t + m(-b + \Delta x)$. We thus have that

$$m(-b) = [1 - p(\Delta t)] \cdot [\Delta t + m(-b)] + p(\Delta t) \cdot [\Delta t + m(-b + \Delta x)]$$

We rearrange this equation so as to construct a difference quotient involving the function m, giving

$$-\frac{1}{p(\Delta t)} = \frac{m(-b + \Delta x) - m(-b)}{\Delta x} \cdot \frac{\Delta x}{\Delta t}$$

$$\approx m'(-b) \cdot \frac{\Delta x}{\Delta t} = \frac{m'(-b)}{\sqrt{\Delta t}} \cdot \frac{\Delta x}{\sqrt{\Delta t}} \tag{6.46}$$

We now consider the value of the expressions in Eq. (6.46) in the limit of $\Delta t \to 0$. We know from Eq. (4.9) that the step probability $p(\Delta t)$ then must tend to $\frac{1}{2}$, and so the left-hand side tends to -2, that is, to a finite, nonzero number. On the right-most side, Δx is of the order $\sqrt{\Delta t}$, so that the ratio of these quantities also converges to a finite, nonzero number. This means that the fraction $\frac{m'(-b)}{\sqrt{\Delta t}}$ must also converge to a finite number, and this in turn clearly requires that $m'(-b) = 0$, for otherwise the right-hand side of Eq. (6.46) would diverge as $\Delta t \to 0$, whereas the left-hand side does not.

In conclusion, then, the boundary conditions for $m(x)$ with a reflecting barrier placed at $-b$ and an absorbing barrier at a are

$$m'(-b) \; = \; 0 \quad \text{and} \quad m(a) = 0 \tag{6.47}$$

6.4.2   Mean First-Passage Times

To illustrate how Eqs. (6.45) and (6.47) are used to find mean first-passage times, let us first consider the standard example of the Wiener process $\mu(x) = \mu, \sigma^2(x) = \sigma^2$, with $b = 0$ as the reflecting barrier and $a > 0$ as the absorbing barrier. With these choices, the general solution of the differential Eq. (6.45) for $m'(x)$ is

$$m'(x) = \left(C + \frac{1}{\mu} \right) \exp\left(-\frac{2\mu}{\sigma^2} x \right) - \frac{1}{\mu} \tag{6.48}$$

and from the boundary condition $m'(0) = 0$ for the reflecting barrier, we immediately deduce that $C = 0$. This implies that $m'(x) < 0$ and so $m(x)$ is strictly decreasing in $x \geq 0$. As expected, the mean first-passage time $E[T \mid X(0) = x]$ will be smaller the closer to the absorbing barrier at a the process starts (Fig. 6.9).

Integrating once more, now using the other boundary condition $m(a) = 0$ from Eq. (6.47), we get for $x \geq 0$

$$m(x) = \frac{a - x}{\mu} - \frac{\sigma^2}{2\mu^2} \cdot \left[\exp\left(-\frac{2\mu x}{\sigma^2} \right) - \exp\left(-\frac{2\mu a}{\sigma^2} \right) \right] \tag{6.49}$$

Defining the auxiliary function $h(z) = z + \frac{\sigma^2}{2\mu} \exp\left(-\frac{2\mu z}{\sigma^2} \right)$, we can write $m(x)$ more compactly as

$$m(x) = \frac{1}{\mu} \cdot [\, h(a) - h(x) \,] \tag{6.50}$$

which forms the counterpart to Eq. (6.36) with two absorbing barriers.

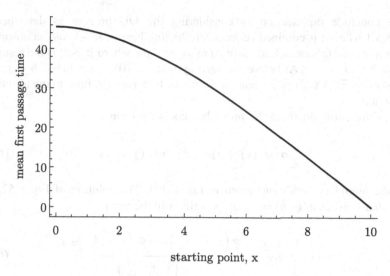

Fig. 6.9 The mean first-passage time (ordinate) as a function of the starting position x (abscissa) for the Wiener process, $\mu(x) = \mu = 0.15$, $\sigma^2(x) = 1$; the reflecting barrier is placed at $b = 0$ and the absorbing barrier at $a = 10$. The line shows the mean first-passage time $m(x)$; see Eq. (6.49). The boundary condition Eq. (6.47) means that $m(x)$ must approach the lower barrier horizontally

Note that when the drift μ is positive, then $x < a$ implies that the second term on the right-hand side of Eq. (6.49), $\frac{\sigma^2}{2\mu^2} \cdot \left[\exp\left(-\frac{2\mu x}{\sigma^2}\right) - \exp\left(-\frac{2\mu a}{\sigma^2}\right) \right]$, is positive. From Exercise 4 of Chap. 4, we know that for a Wiener process with drift $\mu > 0$, the mean first-passage time from x to a single barrier at $a > x$ is equal to the first term on the right-hand side of Eq. (6.49), that is, to $(a - x)/\mu$. Therefore, the second summand represents the "saving" in mean first-passage time due to the presence of a reflecting barrier at $b = 0$, which effectively prevents the Wiener process from wandering off into negative states. Clearly, the mean amount of time saved increases in a and decreases in x, that is, it increases with the distance of the starting point x to the barrier at a.

From Eq. (6.50), it is particularly easy to derive the limit $\mu \to 0$, equal to

$$\lim_{\mu \to 0} m(x) = \frac{a^2 - x^2}{\sigma^2} \tag{6.51}$$

As for the conditional means, the same result is obtained when the differential Eq. (6.45) is solved for $\sigma^2(x) = \sigma^2$ and $\mu(x) = 0$ under the boundary conditions indicated in Eq. (6.47).

Compared to the corresponding result Eq. (6.35), for the mean conditional time to absorption at a, the mean first-passage time is considerably larger when $b = 0$ is a reflecting rather than an absorbing barrier. This corresponds to informal intuition, as in the first case upon reaching $b = 0$, the process continues till it ultimately absorbs at a, which necessarily prolongs the mean first-passage time to a.

We conclude this section by considering the OU process as described in Sect. 5.3.1 when it is confined between a reflecting barrier at $-b$ and an absorbing barrier at a. For this model, we have $\mu(x) = \mu - \beta x$ where $\beta > 0$ is the restoring force and $\sigma^2(x) = \sigma^2$. As before, the starting state is $X(0) = x$, where $-b < x < a$, and $m(x) = \mathsf{E}[T|X(0) = x]$ denotes the mean first-passage time to the absorbing barrier at a.

The differential Eq. (6.45) for $m(x)$ then takes the form

$$\frac{1}{2}\sigma^2 m''(x) + (\mu - \beta x)\, m'(x) = -1 \tag{6.52}$$

with the boundary conditions given in Eq. (6.47). The solution of Eq. (6.52) for $m'(x)$ that satisfies $m'(-b) = 0$ may be written in the form

$$m'(x) = -\frac{2}{\sigma^2} \cdot \frac{\Phi\left(x\left|\frac{\mu}{\beta}, \frac{\sigma^2}{2\beta}\right.\right) - \Phi\left(-b\left|\frac{\mu}{\beta}, \frac{\sigma^2}{2\beta}\right.\right)}{n\left(x\left|\frac{\mu}{\beta}, \frac{\sigma^2}{2\beta}\right.\right)} \tag{6.53}$$

where Φ und n are, respectively, the normal distribution and density function with the indicated mean μ/β and variance $\sigma^2/(2\beta)$. As expected, the function m' is negative so that m decreases as the starting state x increases: $\mathsf{E}[T|X(0) = x]$ will be smaller the closer to the absorbing barrier the OU process starts.

Equation (6.53) cannot be explicitly integrated; we choose the integral of $m'(x)$ such that m satisfies $m(a) = 0$ as required by Eq. (6.47), namely,

$$m(x) = \frac{2}{\sigma^2} \cdot \int_x^a \frac{\Phi\left(v\left|\frac{\mu}{\beta}, \frac{\sigma^2}{2\beta}\right.\right) - \Phi\left(-b\left|\frac{\mu}{\beta}, \frac{\sigma^2}{2\beta}\right.\right)}{n\left(v\left|\frac{\mu}{\beta}, \frac{\sigma^2}{2\beta}\right.\right)}\, dv \tag{6.54}$$

Note that in Eq. (6.54), the starting state x appears as the lower limit of the integral; on differentiating Eq. (6.54), this feature produces the negative sign on the right-hand side of Eq. (6.53).

Figure 6.10 shows the typical course of $m(x)$. The marked asymmetry of $m(x)$ with respect to the midline ($x = 0$) between the barriers shown in Fig. 6.10 means that changes of the starting position to the left of $x = 0$ have relatively little effect. This reflects that $\mu(x)$ increases as x decreases so that in the region $x < 0$, the process reverts swiftly toward $x = 0$. In contrast, changes of the starting position to the right of $x = 0$ have a strong impact which reflects the mean-reverting effect built into the drift component $\mu(x) = \mu - \beta x$ of the OU model. Note that as $b \to \infty$ in Eq. (6.54), we get the one-sided mean first-passage time of the OU process to the barrier at a when starting at $x < a$.

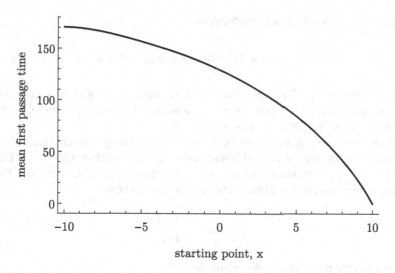

Fig. 6.10 The mean first-passage time (ordinate) as a function of the starting position x (abscissa) for the Ornstein–Uhlenbeck model, $\mu(x) = 0.1 - 0.015x$, $\sigma^2(x) = 1$; the reflecting barrier is placed at $-b = -10$ and the absorbing barrier at $a = 10$. The line shows the mean first-passage time $m(x)$; see Eq. (6.54). The boundary condition Eq. (6.47) means that $m(x)$ must approach the lower barrier horizontally

6.5 Exercises

1. The mean first-passage time $m(x)$ for the Wiener process with absorbing barriers at $b = 0$ and $a > 0$ is given by Eq. (6.13). Show that as $\mu \to 0$, the function $m(x)$ tends to $x(a - x)/\sigma^2$. Confirm that this limit corresponds to the solution of Eq. (6.11) with $\sigma^2(x) = \sigma$ and $\mu(x) = 0$.

2. Based on considerations of symmetry, argue from Eq. (6.37) for the Wiener process with $\mu = 0$ that for the absorption at the lower barrier $b = 0$

$$\mathsf{E}[\mathsf{T}|X(\mathsf{T}) = 0] = \frac{x(2a - x)}{3\sigma^2}$$

Using this result, the previous exercise, and Eq. (6.37), explicitly confirm for this special case the general relation that

$$\mathsf{E}[\mathsf{T}] = \mathsf{E}[\mathsf{T}|X(\mathsf{T}) = a] \cdot \pi_+(x) + \mathsf{E}[\mathsf{T}|X(\mathsf{T}) = 0] \cdot (1 - \pi_+(x))$$

3. By considering the outcome of the first step, argue that for a symmetric discrete random walk with start at x, the mean first-passage time to a barrier satisfies

$$\mathsf{E}[\mathsf{T}|X(0) = x] = m(x) = 1 + \frac{1}{2}\left[m(x + 1) + m(x - 1)\right]$$

Rewriting this equation in the form of

$$\frac{1}{2}\left[m(x+1) - 2m(x) + m(x-1)\right] = -1$$

argue (using, e.g., Eq. (3.5)) that for distant barriers (relative to a single step), this equation tends to $\frac{1}{2}m''(x) = -1$, which is the simplest form of the basic Eq. (6.11) for the drift-free case of $\mu(x) = 0$.

4. Consider diffusion processes between two absorbing barriers placed at $-b$ and a for the special case of homoscedasticity in which $\sigma^2(x) = \sigma^2$. Define $k(x) = \frac{2}{\sigma^2}\int_{-b}^{x}\mu(v)\,dv$ and $H_{\pm}(x) = \int_{-b}^{x}\exp[\pm k(v)]\,dv$. Show that (when these integrals converge) the probability to absorb at a is

$$\pi_+(x) = \frac{H_-(x)}{H_-(a)}$$

and that the mean first-passage time is

$$m(x) = \frac{2}{\sigma^2}\left[\pi_+(x)G(a) - G(x)\right]$$

where $G(x) = \int_{-b}^{x}\exp[-k(v)]\,H_+(v)\,dv$.

5. Use the equations for $\pi_+(x)$ and $m(x)$ from Exercise 4 to confirm the results for the Wiener process with drift and for the regression-type model $\mu(x) = \cot(x)$, $\sigma^2 = 1$.

6. Consider the regression-type diffusion model characterized by $\mu(x) = \cot(x)$, $\sigma^2 = 1$, with a reflecting barrier placed at $-b = \pi/4$ and an absorbing barrier at $a = 3\pi/4$. Use the differential Eq. (6.45) for the mean first-passage time to show that under the boundary conditions Eq. (6.47), we get

$$m(x) = \left(x - \frac{\pi}{4} + \frac{1}{2}\right)\cot(x) + \frac{1+\pi}{2}$$

which satisfies $m'(-b) = 0$ and $m(a) = 0$.

7. Analyze the mean-reverting model characterized by $\mu(x) = \cot(x)$ shown in Fig. 6.3 for the case of $\sigma^2 < 1$. To this end, use numerical routines or a symbolic computer algebra system to solve Eqs. (6.11) and (6.24) for two absorbing barriers. Confirm that for $\sigma^2 < 1$, the mean-reverting effect is enhanced, as would be expected if local chance effects are reduced, and so the drift dynamic shown in Fig. 6.3 becomes more pronounced (see Fig. 6.11).

8. Extending the approach in Sect. 5.5, show that for the expected squared first-passage time, $q(x) = \mathsf{E}[\mathbf{T}^2]$, we have (cf., Eq. (5.40))

$$\sigma^2(x)\,q''(x) + \mu(x)\,q'(x) = -2m(x)$$

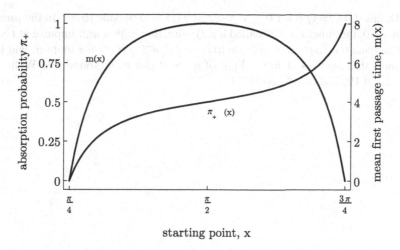

starting point, x

Fig. 6.11 Mean first-passage time (right ordinate) and absorption probability (left ordinate) for the diffusion model $\mu(x) = \cot(x)$, $\sigma^2(x) = 0.25$. The peaked curve shows the mean first-passage time $m(x) = \mathsf{E}[T|X(0) = x]$ as a function of the start position x (abscissa) of the process between the absorbing barriers at $-b = \pi/4$ and $a = 3\pi/4$. The increasing curve shows the probability $\pi_+(x)$ to absorb at the upper barrier a. Due to the strong mean-reverting effect, variations of the start point x in the middle region have little effect on the absorption probability and mean first-passage time. Compare to the corresponding results for $\sigma^2 = 1$ shown in Fig. 6.4.

Note that in order to solve this equation for $q(x)$, we first need to find $m(x)$ from Eq. (6.11).

Show that for the Wiener process with drift μ and variance σ^2 between an absorbing barrier at a and a reflecting barrier at $b = 0$, we get for the variance of the first-passage time

$$\mathsf{Var}(\mathbf{T} \mid X(0) = x) = q(x) - m^2(x) = \frac{1}{(k\mu)^2} \left[w(a) - w(x) \right]$$

$$\text{where} \quad w(u) = 2ku + \exp(-ku) \cdot \left[4 + 4ku + \exp(-ku) \right]$$

and $k = 2\mu/\sigma^2$. Show that this expression tends in the limit of $\mu \to 0$ to

$$\mathsf{Var}(\mathbf{T} \mid X(0) = x) = \frac{2}{3\sigma^4} (a^4 - x^4)$$

9. Using the differential equation for $q(x)$ in Exercise 8, show that for the Wiener process with $\mu = 0$ and variance σ^2 between two absorbing barriers at 0 and at a, the variance of the first-passage time is

$$\mathsf{Var}(\mathbf{T} \mid X(0) = x) = q(x) - m^2(x) = \frac{1}{3\sigma^4} x \cdot (a - x) \cdot \left[x^2 + (a - x)^2 \right]$$

Compare this result to the corresponding result of Exercise 8.

10. Define $f(t) = 1/h$ for $0 \leq t \leq h$ and $f(t) = 0$ outside $[0, h]$. In the limit of $h \to 0$, the function f is called a $\delta(t)$−function with a unit impulse at $t = 0$. Compute the Laplace transform $u(s) = \int_0^\infty e^{-st} f(t)dt$ for finite h, and then show that $u(s) \to 1$ in the limit of $h \to 0$ (for background, see Wylie and Barrett 1995, ch.s 9.5 and 10.11).

Chapter 7
Applications of Random Walk and Diffusion Models in the Life and Behavioral Sciences

The following sections present some of the more elementary and straightforward applications of random walk and diffusion models in the life and behavioral sciences. Our intention here is to convey basic concepts and to focus on central, original ideas on which these applications are based, not to scrutinize technical details of the examples discussed. The literature on diffusion models of, for example, animal movement or human decision and choice behavior both contain several thousand original studies. It is, therefore, evident that our review is necessarily highly selective and simplified; however, references are given for each area to follow up on more detailed or complex aspects. It seems remarkable that often the same type of model is analyzed and applied in quite different substantive areas, using distinct jargon, terminology, notation, and even formalisms. This impressive fact certainly suggests that random walk and diffusion models capture fundamental aspects of reality acting at very different scales and levels of research, but it also can make it difficult to translate important insights from one area to another.

7.1 Stephen J. Gould: The Spread of Excellence

In 1996, the well-known paleontologist Stephen J. Gould proposed a general theory that aims to explain, among other things, why an overall improvement in fitness or design may nevertheless lead to a decrement in many performance-related contexts. In fact, Gould argued that overall improvements are often the immediate cause of such decrements; his main example to illustrate this relation comes from baseball and concerns the decline of the batting average. His arguments, which clearly generalize to many contexts other than baseball as well, are mainly statistical in nature and may be easily explained in terms of diffusion models involving a reflecting barrier.

© Springer Nature Switzerland AG 2022
W. Schwarz, *Random Walk and Diffusion Models*,
https://doi.org/10.1007/978-3-031-12100-5_7

The batting average of a player in baseball is the relative proportion of times at bat in which he hits the ball. Gould documents that from the early to the late twentieth century, outstanding averages (such as a value of 0.400) have become more and more rare. At first sight, this finding seems puzzling because in general during that period, baseball has become much more professional—why, then, are outstanding performances (such as an average of 0.400) less, not more, frequent?

Gould interprets the batting process as the result of a competition between the batter and the pitcher. In effect, the ability of the pitcher to throw the ball is pitted against the hitting skill of the batter so that the batting process takes the general form of a paired comparison. This notion is one key feature in his account of decreasing top batting averages.

Gould's central ideas essentially refer to the dynamics as seen in simple diffusion processes involving a single reflecting barrier (cf., Sect. 4.3). As reviewed in detail by Gould (1996, ch. 9), in the top leagues, there has been a massive overall improvement in the player's individual performance level across time, due to better training, an optimized lifestyle, and also an increase in relevant body measures. In diffusion terms, this general trend may be represented by a positive drift, toward increasing values representing higher performance. Gould argues that at the same time, there exists an upper performance limit—called by him "the right wall"— that for biomechanical reasons cannot possibly be exceeded. For example, despite all improvements in sports science and nutrition, man will never be able to fly. Likewise, the time for the transmission of neural signals from the eye to the brain of a batter plus the time for issuing appropriate motor commands steering his arm movements will never reduce to, say, 10 ms. Gould's central concept of a "right wall" may be represented in diffusion terms as a reflecting barrier to the right.

In Gould's model, the idealized process of how top baseball developed consists of three successive stages, which can be interpreted in analogy to the three phases depicted in Fig. 4.7. At a first stage, there will be just a small group of amateurish players who all have similarly low performance levels. During this stage, corresponding to the left panel in Fig. 4.7, not only is the overall performance average low but also the performance variance is small, as all players compete at a similar, low level. As shown in the middle panel of Fig. 4.7, after some time, considerable differences between competing players will evolve. This implies that during this second stage, excellent players will often compete against players with fairly limited skills. Because batting averages essentially reflect the outcome of many paired batter-pitcher comparisons, it is during this phase that there exist top players who are far ahead of the average level, and it is this constellation that leads to outstanding batting averages like 0.400. At a final stage (present-day baseball, corresponding to the right panel of Fig. 4.7), essentially all baseball players in the top leagues are high-performance professionals, which means that the average difference among players is much lower than during the preceding intermediate stage.

These observations are summarized in Fig. 7.1 which shows the increasing mean but first increasing then decreasing standard deviation of a Wiener process with positive drift in the presence of a reflecting barrier at $a = 100$. The positive drift

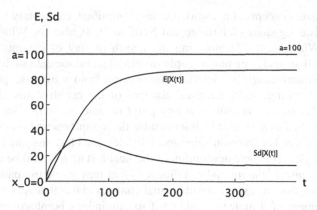

Fig. 7.1 The mean $E[X(t)]$ and standard deviation $Sd[X(t)]$ (ordinate) of a Wiener process starting at $x_0 = 0$ (origin of the ordinate) with drift $\mu = 1$ and $\sigma = 5$ in the presence of a reflecting barrier at $a = 100$ (shown as upper horizontal line) as a function of time, t (abscissa). Given that the drift is directed toward the reflecting barrier at $a = 100$, the mean $E[X(t)]$ increases with time. In contrast, the standard deviation $Sd[X(t)]$ initially increases but then decreases toward its asymptotic level, equal to $\sigma^2/(2\mu)$. Gould's model considers performance measures based on competitions of the paired comparison type, which thus essentially reflect the variance (or Sd) among the competitors at any time

reflects the improvement of mean performance with time across all players, and the reflecting barrier corresponds to Gould's "right wall". Performance measures based on competitions of the paired comparison type essentially reflect the *variance* at any time among the competitors. If one considers picking at random two players out of the population during the final stage, then their difference in performance level will on average be relatively small, which translates into batting averages clearly below 0.400.

In short, in Gould's model, performance in contexts where competition follows paired comparison designs essentially reflects the variance, not the mean, across the participants competing at any time. Evidently, very similar trends are seen in many other contexts where the times of "towering figures and legendary heroes" are long gone. To take an obvious example, in the 1907 chess world champion final, Emanuel Lasker beat Frank Marshall by 8-7-0, an outcome that would be considered inconceivable in present-day world-class chess.

7.2   Modeling First Hitting Times

George Alex Whitmore did pioneering work in the application of diffusion models to account for the dynamics of a wide variety of real-world processes which before him seemed not amenable to quantitative modeling at a microscopic level.

Various main concepts of his work are, in a simplified, elementary form, clearly present in his early study (Whitmore and Neufeld 1970; also see Whitmore 1975; Eaton and Whitmore 1977) modeling the length of stay of patients in hospital units. Rather than analyzing macroscopic structural and static data such as actuarial records, Whitmore sought to describe this process from a microscopic real-time perspective, focusing on the temporal changes of the health status of individual patients. In his conceptualization, at any point in time, an individual has a state of health, denoted as $h(t)$, that is described by the symptoms and prognosis and is measured as his or her score on some specially designed test or some combination of such tests. Any complete description of the health state h would be exceedingly complex. Because of the myriad of influences that may cause the patient's health level to deviate from its expected path, actual changes in health level can be likened to the movement of a molecule subjected to continuous bombardment by other molecules—the standard assumptions described in Chap. 3 leading to the normal distribution and the Wiener process.

Let $h(t)$ denote the level of an individual's health on this scale at time t—in essence, $h(t)$ describes the course of the individual's health level over the time period considered. If large (small) values of h denote good (poor) health, a basic assumption is that when h falls to the critical level a, then the individual in question is admitted to hospital for treatment and care; in Fig. 7.2, this happens at time t_1. If, and when, h returns for the first time to the higher level $b > a$, the individual has recovered and is discharged from the unit; in Fig. 7.2, this happens at time t_2. Thus, the time $t_2 - t_1$ it takes $h(t)$ to move from a to b is the patient's length of stay; in Whitmore's conceptualization, it corresponds to the first-passage time to b

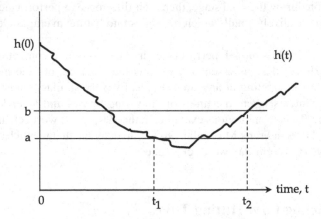

Fig. 7.2 The Whitmore model of the length of stay of patients in hospital units. Ordinate, health level h; abscissa, time, t. The path $h(t)$ denotes the level of an individual's health. At time t_1, the health level h falls to a critical level a, and the individual is admitted to hospital for treatment and care. When h returns for the first time (t_2) to the higher level $b > a$, the individual is discharged from the unit. Thus, the first-passage time $t_2 - t_1$ from a (admittance at t_1) to b (discharge at t_2) represents the patient's length of stay

(discharge) starting from a (admission); its distribution corresponds to the density of Eq. (4.23).

In this model, a and b are important policy parameters. The greater the difference $b - a$, the greater must be the improvement in a patient's health before he or she is released from the hospital. Also, the larger the a, the more quickly will individuals with deteriorating health be admitted to the hospital. For an inpatient, the drift parameter μ of the process then measures the propensity for getting well. The variance parameter σ^2 measures the extent to which a person's health might depart from its expected level. Thus, an individual with a large volatility parameter σ^2 is likely to show wide health state swings over short periods of time.

Whitmore (1976) reviews several management applications of this *first hitting model*, leading to the inverse Gaussian distribution Eq. (4.23), such as price development, business survival times, or the length of periods of unemployment and employment. The latter example is studied in considerable detail in Whitmore (1979), based on the following intuitive and elegant conceptualization. As an employee absorbs day-to-day experiences related to his or her work, the level of job attachment $X(t)$ is bound to fluctuate over time. The critical level of attachment— below which one gives notice—defines the so-called separation threshold. The first-passage time to this separation threshold then defines the employee's completed length of service with the organization. In this model, the level of job attachment $X(t)$ is assumed to be a Wiener process; if it reaches the separation threshold, the employee will quit. Denoting $X(0) = x_0 > 0$ as the initial attachment to the job, Whitmore applied this model to several detailed data sets and discussed how changes in the various model parameters (μ, σ^2, x_0) will influence the probability of quitting the job and the distribution of the completed length of service. He also discusses tractable mixing distributions for the parameters of the implied inverse Gaussian distributions, which arise when different employees of a cohort are characterized by different model parameters (μ, σ^2, x_0).

A closely related example of diffusion-based modeling of real-world processes is Lancaster's (1972) account of the duration of a strike. In his conceptualization, a strike is interpreted as a process of bargaining and concession between two parties. More generally, Lancaster's account is a model of conflict resolution, negotiation, bargaining, and settlement, as characterized by dispute, demand, and offer. These demands and offers will change as experience accumulates and expectations are revised, and work will be resumed when the management provides an offer consistent with the workers' current demand, that is, when at some point in time t, the difference between offer $O(t)$ and demand $D(t)$ first reaches a threshold of agreement. In this view, the critical variable at any time t is defined as offer minus demand, $X(t) = O(t) - D(t)$, which at the begin of the conflict (when the demand is higher than the offer) takes negative values. Given the multitudinous components influencing $X(t)$ at any time, it is not unreasonable to assume that $X(t)$ forms a Wiener process with drift μ and variance σ^2; in this interpretation, μ is the mean drift to settlement per time unit (e.g., working day), reflecting increased offers and/or lowered demands. The strike is over when for the first time the disagreement $X(t)$ reaches an agreement threshold. For example, the variables O and D might refer to an hourly wage; in other cases, the difference $O - D$ between the parties in a dispute can be some more complex hypothetical or postulated construct. Lancaster (1972) fitted his model to strikes in the UK and found (with t measured in days) for different industries estimates in the order of $\mu = 0.2$ and $\sigma = 0.7$, which implies the mean strike duration is about 5 days, with a standard deviation of about 8 days. Across the strikes analyzed, he found the ratio of σ/μ to stay remarkably close to about 4. One interpretation of Lancaster's finding is that all industries have similar σ/μ ratios but that the agreement threshold varies across industries.

An original application of first hitting models is by Tshiswaka-Kashalala and Koch (2017) who studied, for women living in the Democratic Republic of Congo, the time to first childbirth and the ability of contraception to extend that time. Specifically, they consider a Wiener process starting at $x_0 > 0$ that represents the time-varying subjective continuation value for a given woman of postponing childbearing by contraception at time t. The time of conception leading to the first birth is the moment when the continuation value process has first dropped to zero, that is, the first-passage time to $x = 0$.

Whitmore's concept of first hitting times has subsequently been generalized to incorporate various observational schemes and covariates, as in standard regression-like data structures. Much of the work on first hitting time models is carefully summarized and reviewed in detail by Whitmore, Ramsay and Aaron (2012), Lee and Whitmore (2006), and Aalen, Borgan and Gjessing (2008).

7.3   Correlated Random Walks: Generalizations and Applications

Correlated random walks were first described and analyzed by Taylor (1922) and Fürth (1920), whose astute paper presents an elementary and elegant analysis. Naturally, the simplest form of correlated random walks described in Sect. 2.4.1 has been generalized very considerably; and these models have been applied in a surprising variety of substantive contexts of which we can only mention a few characteristic or influential examples.

A profound generalization of correlated random walks is to permit different persistence strengths (in the sense of Sect. 2.4) following an upward (p_0) and a downward (p_1) step. The basic transition matrix then becomes

$$\mathbf{X}_{n+1}$$

$$\begin{array}{c} \qquad\quad - \qquad\quad + \\ \mathbf{X}_n \quad \begin{array}{c} - \\ + \end{array} \begin{bmatrix} p_0 & 1 - p_0 \\ 1 - p_1 & p_1 \end{bmatrix} \end{array} \qquad (7.1)$$

The symmetric case, as defined by the matrix (2.32) in Chap. 2, is the special case $p_0 = p_1 = p$. In essence, Eq. (7.1) defines a two-state Markov chain with general transition probabilities whose states refer to the possible direction of each step. The behavior of the asymmetric model differs considerably from that of the symmetric model in several ways. For example, asymmetric persistence will add a systematic drift component to the process, meaning that $E[X_n]$ will no longer remain bounded as $n \to \infty$.

One important application of this model is the binomial sampling scheme when the two outcomes per step are success and failure and their probabilities depend on the outcome of the previous trial. The model has first been analyzed in full by Gabriel (1959) and has been applied by him to study the persistence of dry and rainy days at a given location. As reviewed by Hanneken and Franceschetti (1998), models equivalent to the asymmetric correlated random walk have been used to analyze cell migration, polymer folding, diffusion in crystals, heartbeat behavior, and human posture. These authors give a clear and straightforward derivation of many detailed (including exact distributional) aspects of the asymmetric correlated random walk and discuss some of its applications. The extension of asymmetric correlated random walks to diffusion models based on the limiting process described in Chap. 3 is treated very clearly by Pottier (1996).

7.4   Random Walk and Diffusion Models of Animal Movement

As briefly reviewed in Chap. 1, animal movement has been a field in which random walk and diffusion models have been applied since early in the twentieth century. Correlated random walks are sometimes used as a simplified model of persistent movement processes; in fact, the first publication on correlated random walks (Fürth 1920) successfully used this model to account for the distance traveled by paramecia in a water solution as a function of time. However, animal movement processes are typically measured in two (or even three) dimensions, whereas the spatial scale of correlated random walks as described by Eq. (7.1) is genuinely uni-dimensional.

Thus, more general models take the notion of a "walk" in the more usual meaning in which the successive steps arise in a two-dimensional plane. A straightforward approach to model two-dimensional animal movement is due to Broadbent and Kendall (1953). In their model, the successive spatial displacements in each discrete time step (e.g., from one registration time point to the next) are independent realizations from a bivariate normal distribution. In the simplest case of completely random movement, both means and the correlation of this normal are zero, with identical variance σ^2 in both directions. Of course, the successive spatial positions occupied by this walk will still be highly correlated as they contain many common summands.

Denoting the animal's position after n steps as (x_n, y_n), the x_n and y_n are independent and are each the sum of n zero-mean normal random variables, all with the same variance, σ^2. This means that the coordinates x_n and y_n are independent normal variables, with mean zero and variance $n\sigma^2$. Denoting the start of the movement as the origin $(0,0)$, the expected position after n steps is still $(0,0)$, and the squared displacement $\mathbf{R}_n^2 = x_n^2 + y_n^2$ is the sum of two independent χ_1^2 variables, each scaled (i.e., multiplied) by $n\sigma^2$. Two independent χ_1^2 variables add to χ_2^2, which is an exponential random variable with an expectation equal to 2. Therefore, $\mathbf{R}_n^2 = n\sigma^2 \chi_2^2$, and so the expected squared displacement after n steps is $\mathsf{E}[\mathbf{R}_n^2] = 2n\sigma^2$. In fact, the probability that after n steps the animal is within a circle of radius r centered on the origin of the movement is equal to $\mathsf{P}(\mathbf{R}_n \leq r) = \mathsf{P}(\mathbf{R}_n^2 \leq r^2) = \mathsf{P}[\chi_2^2 \leq r^2/(n\sigma^2)] = 1 - \exp(-\frac{r^2}{2n\sigma^2})$. Thus, the radial distance $\mathbf{R}_n$ follows the so-called Rayleigh distribution; for example, its mean is $\mathsf{E}[\mathbf{R}_n] = \sigma\sqrt{n\pi/2}$. Together with the result about the mean squared displacement, it then follows that $\mathsf{Var}[\mathbf{R}_n] = n\sigma^2(2 - \pi/2)$. For example, the mean and standard deviation of the displacement $\mathbf{R}_n$ after n steps should generally be proportional to each other, the coefficient of variation being close to one-half.

In many situations, an unrealistic feature of this model is the lack of spatial persistence across successive steps, once the animal has chosen a targeted direction. Thus, as a potentially more realistic model of animal movement consider that the walk starts at point $\mathbf{S}_0 = (0, 0)$. In each discrete step n, a turning angle $\boldsymbol{\alpha}_n$ and a step length $\mathbf{L}_n$ are chosen at random according to some joint distribution $g(\alpha, L)$. Then a straight-line step of length $\mathbf{L}_n$ is executed such that the direction of the walk *relative to the previous step* is changed by $\boldsymbol{\alpha}_n$ degrees. For example, if $\boldsymbol{\alpha}_n = 0$, then the process continues in the same direction as before, and for $\boldsymbol{\alpha}_n = \pi$, it reverses to the opposite direction.

As shown in Fig. 7.3, starting at $(0, 0)$, the first step will increment the walk to a point (x_1, y_1) with coordinates $\Delta x_1 = \mathbf{L}_1 \cdot \cos(\boldsymbol{\alpha}_1)$ and $\Delta y_1 = \mathbf{L}_1 \cdot \sin(\boldsymbol{\alpha}_1)$. From there, the next step induces a horizontal increment $\Delta x_2 = x_2 - x_1$ equal to $\Delta x_2 = \mathbf{L}_2 \cdot \cos(\boldsymbol{\alpha}_1 + \boldsymbol{\alpha}_2)$. Similarly, the vertical increment $\Delta y_2 = y_2 - y_1$ is equal to $\Delta y_2 = \mathbf{L}_2 \cdot \sin(\boldsymbol{\alpha}_1 + \boldsymbol{\alpha}_2)$. Together, the coordinates of the second point (x_2, y_2) are equal to $(x_1 + \Delta x_2, y_1 + \Delta y_2)$. Continuing in the same manner, the position (x_n, y_n) of the walk after n steps is given by the summed partial increments Δ in x and y,

$$x_n = \sum_{i=1}^{n} \mathbf{L}_i \cdot \cos(\sum_{j=1}^{i} \boldsymbol{\alpha}_j) \quad \text{and} \quad y_n = \sum_{i=1}^{n} \mathbf{L}_i \cdot \sin(\sum_{j=1}^{i} \boldsymbol{\alpha}_j)$$

In effect, the primary summation process of the walk refers to the successive turning angles $\boldsymbol{\alpha}_i$. Based on the partial sums $\sum_{j=1}^{i} \boldsymbol{\alpha}_j$, the coordinates of the walk are then given as indicated. The walk is highly correlated because the summed angles defining two successive positions carry many identical components, leading to a high step-to-step correlation. The expected squared distance from the origin

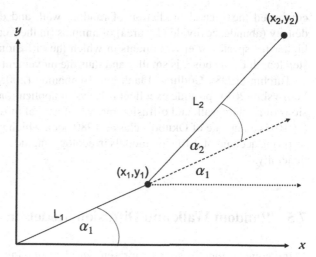

Fig. 7.3 Correlated random walk in two dimensions: in each step, a turning angle α, measured relative to the previous step, and a step length L are chosen. Abscissa x and ordinate y represent the coordinates of the plane in which the animal moves

after n steps can be derived from Euler's identity (Stewart 2012) in a fairly straightforward manner (Exercise 1); for details and explicit results, see Kareiva and Shigesada (1983) and Skellam (1973).

The model depicted in Fig. 7.3 is quite general and flexible. The simple correlated random walk, as defined in Sect. 2.4 by Eq. (2.32), is the rather special case in which all steps L_n have unit length, and all turning angles equal, with probability p, either $0°$ (a persistent continuation) or, with probability $1 - p$, $180°$ (an about-face). Similarly, if the turning angle is either 0 or $180°$ with equal probability, and all steps have unit length, then the simple symmetric random walk of Sect. 2.1 results. In both of these cases, the path of the animal is restricted to one dimension, that is, it walks along a line. On the other hand, the model is able to predict tortuous movement patterns as well. For example, if the turning angle distribution is closely centered on $45°$ and the step lengths are not too variable, then the path of the animal approximates an octagon, returning roughly to its origin after eight steps. In many applications, the targeted direction of the animal would correspond to the x−axis, and the mean turning angle would be zero. In this case, the animal will in expectation home in on the target direction but will oscillate around a straight-line path to a degree that depends on the spread of the angle distribution.

Kareiva and Shigesada (1983) analyzed the flight sequences of over 200 small whites, a butterfly species. A single step of the random walk was defined as the transition from one landing site to the next. In the range of up to 14 steps, the mean squared displacement corresponded closely to the prediction of the model in Fig. 7.3. On a different spatial and temporal scale, Bergman, Schaefer and Luttich (2000) used satellite telemetry to investigate long-distance movements of reindeer. On a monthly time scale, they observed excellent correspondence between the mean squared displacements of caribou and the predictions of the model shown in Fig. 7.3. Over an annual cycle, the model overestimated the displacement through time, indicating a propensity for site fidelity. Schultz et al. (2017) tested and confirmed the general prediction of random walk and diffusion models that the density (abundance divided by area) of animals (in their case, butterflies) should be higher for species or environments in which the diffusion coefficient, or the mean step length E[L] above, is smaller and thus the movement is slower.

Turchin (1998), Codling, Plank and Benhamou (2008), and Lewis, Maini and Petrovskii (2013) provide excellent reviews of applications, limitations, and extensions of random walk and diffusion models of animal movement. Okubo and Levin (2010) is an update of Okubo's classic 1980 book which provides an ingenious and inspiring account of diffusion models in ecology, including animal movement, more generally.

7.5   Random Walk and Diffusion Models in Sports

Many competitions in sports represent an ideal playing ground for random walk and diffusion models: their scores are genuinely quantitative, and the manner in which they change over time defines a stochastic process whose characteristics are of considerable interest.

A seminal diffusion-based contribution to this area is the work of Stern (1994). Using basketball as one example, he described the within-match dynamics by focusing on the home team lead, that is, on the running score difference of the home minus the away team. Stern modeled the home team lead during the course of a match as a Wiener diffusion process, with drift μ and variance σ^2. The drift μ in this model measures the home team advantage—by how much the home team lead increases (if $\mu > 0$) on average per time unit—whereas σ describes the variation around this mean. In contrast to sports with a slow transferral of play and few scoring events, basketball is characterized by rapid changes and a high scoring pace. It is thus a plausible candidate sport of which it seems a priori reasonable to expect that the assumptions of Stern's model are met to a fair approximation. The model implies that the score difference is normally distributed with mean and variance proportional to the time in the play. If the match lasts for a total of t time units (e.g., $t = 40$ minutes, in most basketball leagues), the final score difference should be normally distributed with mean μt and variance $\sigma^2 t$, which means that the probability of a home team win (i.e., a positive final score difference) is equal to $\Phi\left(\frac{\mu}{\sigma}\sqrt{t}\right)$. For example, the winning probability of the better team increases with playing time; shorter match durations provide the weaker team with an opportunity to win against the odds.

Stern (1994) tested these assumptions and predictions empirically in considerable detail by partitioning each of the results of matches of professional basketball teams into four separate quarter results. He found the changes of the result in separate quarters to be independent, nearly identically distributed, and the normal quantile plots to be very nearly linear. Stern also demonstrated that the continuous diffusion approximation of the necessarily discrete score changes was generally excellent and estimated μ (using 1 min as a time unit) to be close to 0.1 and σ

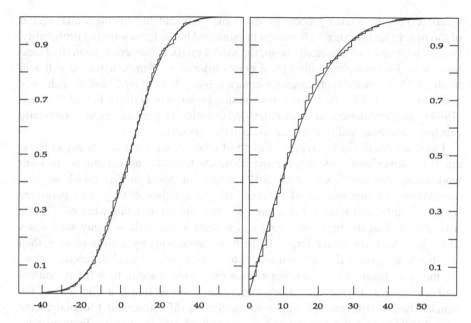

Fig. 7.4 The left panel shows the empirical distribution function (ordinate) of the final difference scores (abscissa) for 323 basketball matches ($t = 40$) analyzed. The smooth line is the cumulative normal distribution function (mean 4.11, standard deviation 15) predicted by Stern's (1994) diffusion model with $\mu = 0.103$ and $\sigma = 2.35$. The right panel shows the empirical distribution function (ordinate) of the maximal home team lead (abscissa) for the same matches. The smooth line is the cumulative distribution function predicted by the diffusion model, using the same parameter estimates as in the left panel

to be close to 2. Thus, at the end of a 40-min match, the mean home team lead would be $\mu t = 4$ points, with a standard deviation $\sigma \sqrt{t} = 2\sqrt{40} \approx 13$; for these values, the probability of a home team win is about 56.3%. An example of the close fit of the model to final score differences is shown in the left panel of Fig. 7.4 for 323 matches of a professional basketball league.

In many statistical analyses of competitive team sport matches, the final score is the variable of major interest. However, individual sport matches also unfold as a dynamical process over time which ultimately leads up to the end result. Approaches based on stochastic processes seek to address the time course of the score change dynamics. A very attractive feature of Stern's (1994) model is that it enables us to go beyond mere end-result statistics. More specifically, Stern was interested in the conditional probability that the home team will win, given the score difference after $0 \leq u < t$ minutes in the game was equal to $X(u) = x$. In his model, this conditional probability clearly corresponds to

$$P[X(t) > 0 | X(u) = x] = \Phi\left(\frac{x + \mu(t - u)}{\sigma\sqrt{t - u}}\right)$$

where $X(t)$ is the Wiener process for the home team lead and t is the total duration of the match; for $u = 0$, $x = 0$, we get the standard home team winning probability. For the parameter values cited above, the model predicts that even when the home team was, for example, behind by 2 points after $u = 5$ min, it would still win in about 55.0% of all such cases. In contrast, being behind by 2 points with only 5 min to go ($u = 35$), the home team winning probability is down to 36.9%. Stern (1994) compared these and similar detailed quantitative predictions systematically to a large data base and found them to be highly accurate.

Using the results in Exercises 13 to 15 of Chap. 4, we can carry Stern's (1994) analysis further and may ask for the distribution of the maximum home team lead during any match (Schwarz 2012). The right panel in Fig. 7.4 shows that the maximum home team lead observed in 323 matches is very well predicted by Stern's diffusion model. For example, when the home team wins by 72−68, it is obvious that the maximum lead was at least 4, but will in many such cases likely have been somewhat larger. If the home team wins by a wide margin, then intuitively we expect the maximum lead to be close to the final difference score. On the other hand, if the home team loses by a wide margin, then the maximum lead will often not have been much larger than zero, as it was at the start of the match. These considerations suggest to use Stern's diffusion model to analyze the joint distribution of the maximum home team lead and the final difference score (Schwarz 2012). Figure 7.5 shows that the diffusion model predicts the empirical relation between these two variables quite well.

Some limitations and shortcomings of the diffusion model may also be noted. For example, Berger and Pope (2011) analyzed all NBA matches from 1993 to 2009 and found that home teams that are behind by one point at half time actually won the match slightly more frequently (58.2%) than home teams leading by one point at the same stage (57.1%). The diffusion model predicts that home teams leading by one point at half time should be more, not less, likely to win the match than home teams trailing by one point. Berger and Pope reason that relative to being slightly ahead, being slightly behind can actually increase motivation and performance, so that trailing teams play better to come back.

Any realistic analysis would certainly have to account for effects related to the strength of the individual teams. For example, we may interpret the difference process in Stern's model as arising from two (possibly correlated) diffusion processes characterizing each team separately; in the simplest case, the net drift μ might be interpreted as the difference $\mu = \mu_h - \mu_a$ of the strength characterizing the home and the away team. Thus, one might relate the drift rate μ_h, μ_a characterizing each team to a linear predictor of relevant regressors via a suitable link function, as in standard generalized linear models (Agresti 2013). Recent results and analyses related to Stern's diffusion model are presented, for example, by Polson and Stern (2015), Chen and Fan (2018), or Gabel and Redner (2012); the *Journal of Quantitative Analysis in Sports* is a major source of random walk and diffusion applications in sports.

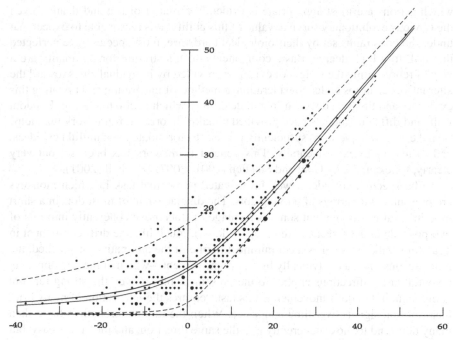

Fig. 7.5 The joint distribution of the maximal home team lead (ordinate) and the final difference score (abscissa) for 323 professional basketball matches. The match whose real-time history is shown in Fig. 1.2 appears at coordinates (4|19). Double and triple data points are indicated by proportionately larger circles. The thick middle line shows the conditional mean maximal home team lead, given the final score; the thinner line slightly below is the corresponding conditional median. The two broken lines show the conditional 5% and 95% quantiles

7.6   Random Walk and Diffusion Models of Animal Decision-Making

7.6.1   Sequential Sampling Models of Neuronal Activity in Perceptual Decision-Making

According to a view made popular by Hermann von Helmholtz (1878; for a more recent version, see Gregory 2015), the brains of animals face a fundamental statistical decision problem: to infer the unknown state of the outer world on the basis of noisy sensory evidence and to select on the basis of these inferences the most appropriate course of action. This noisy sensory evidence comes in the form of time-varying firing (depolarization) rates of neurons in specific brain regions: different neurons and different brain areas respond selectively, with graded intensity, to specific aspects of the outer world. It is this selectivity that enables the animal to construct an internal representation of its environment. The ability of an animal to draw the right conclusions about the state of the world surrounding it and to decide which actions are most appropriate is evidently a matter of life and death. Given the obvious evolutionary survival value of this ability, it is reasonable to expect that under the constraints set by their biological hardware, most species have perfected this task to a high degree. Basic components in this striving for optimality are a way of representing the weight of evidence provided by individual clues toward the alternative scenarios under consideration, a method of integrating and updating this evidence, and finally a decision rule to determine which action to choose. Random walk and diffusion models have provided a major theoretical framework that helps to make research questions sufficiently precise, to formulate meaningful new ideas, and to test them experimentally. This general framework has been set out very clearly, for example, by Gold and Shadlen (2001, 2007) or Schall (2001).

To be specific, consider a well-investigated perceptual task in which monkeys are presented with arrays of moving dots. The displacement of most dots in a short time interval is random, but some percentage of dots move coherently into one of two possible target directions (e.g., up or down), much like the drift component in a random walk. As soon as a commitment to one of the alternatives is reached, the monkey must indicate—typically by an eye movement—which of the two opposing potential target directions applies to the present display. Given the strong random component in the dot's movements, this task requires the integration of many brief local motion signals over time and space. When the motion strength is high, then many dots tend to move coherently into the same direction, and the task is easy, but when the coherence is low, the task is quite difficult. The firing rate of neurons in the middle temporal (MT) area of the brain of primates is finely tuned to the direction of visual movement. Thus, it is the neural activity of neurons in brain area MT which represents the encoded, noisy evidence that the animal must integrate and interpret to decide, for example, between upward (s_1) and downward motion (s_0).

Gold and Shadlen (2001, 2007) presented an influential model, backed by considerable neurophysiological evidence, of how animals arrive at these decisions. During any short time period, each neuron (or pool of similar neurons) has a discharge distribution that is normal with mean μ_1 for motion in its preferred orientation and with mean $\mu_0 < \mu_1$ for motion in the opposite direction. It seems plausible that the sensory evidence the animal is using is the firing rate x of movement-sensitive neurons with preferred upright orientation, so that strong (weak) activation indicates upward (downward) movement. An optimal rule for the animal would be to contrast the posterior probability of the upward vs. downward motion signal, given this evidence,

$$\frac{p(s_1|x)}{p(s_0|x)} = \frac{f(x|s_1)}{f(x|s_0)} \cdot \frac{p(s_1)}{p(s_0)}$$

where $p(s_1)$ and $p(s_0)$ are the prior probabilities of upward and downward movement. In statistical terminology, the posterior odds of an upward movement are the likelihood ratio times the prior odds. In effect, this relation suggests that on the basis of the firing rate x, the animal might decide in favor of an upward movement if the likelihood ratio exceeds a certain threshold set by the prior probabilities. Theoretically, then, the likelihood ratio of the firing rate of neurons under upward vs. downward directions of motion might represent a critical quantity in neural computations. At first sight, it seems remote and biologically implausible that brains solve simple perceptual decisions by doing computations akin to abstract statistical decision theory. However, Gold and Shadlen (2001, 2007) provided biologically plausible arguments how these computations could possibly be neuronally implemented in a simple and stable manner.

Inserting the normal density and taking the logarithm, the log likelihood ratio is seen to be

$$\ln \frac{f(x|s_1)}{f(x|s_0)} = \frac{\mu_1 - \mu_0}{\sigma^2} \left(x - \frac{\mu_1 + \mu_0}{2} \right)$$

For example, a large positive activation $x \gg \mu_1$ from an upward-oriented neuron constitutes strong evidence in favor of the upward direction; if the activation x falls just in between μ_0 and μ_1, then the evidence is even, and the log likelihood ratio is zero. Gold and Shadlen suggest that an adaptive solution to reduce the complexity of likelihood ratio computations is to incorporate a second neuron (or pool of neurons) which responds maximally to downward motion.

In our example, the responses y of these so-called anti-neurons have a normal density g, with a higher mean of μ_1 for their preferred downward motion and with a lower mean of μ_0 for upward motion. On a similar calculation as before, we then get for the log likelihood ratio favoring upward motion from the output provided by the anti-neurons

$$\ln \frac{g(y|s_1)}{g(y|s_0)} = \frac{\mu_0 - \mu_1}{\sigma^2} \left(y - \frac{\mu_0 + \mu_1}{2} \right) = \frac{\mu_1 - \mu_0}{\sigma^2} \left(-y + \frac{\mu_1 + \mu_0}{2} \right)$$

A large positive output y from an anti-neuron represents strong evidence in favor of the downward direction. Combining (adding) the evidence conveyed by both types of neurons, we get for the total log likelihood ratio λ favoring the upward motion after observing the firing rates x and y

$$\lambda(x, y) = \frac{\mu_1 - \mu_0}{\sigma^2} (x - y)$$

The expression for $\lambda(x, y)$ shows that combining the evidence of opposing neurons leads to a stable, biologically implementable rule: simply register the difference of the activity of neurons with preferred upward vs. downward direction. If for a given neuron and interval the firing rate is normally distributed, then the difference signal $x - y$ is normally distributed, too. For upward motion, the mean of the difference signal $x - y$ will be $\mu_1 - \mu_0 > 0$, and for downward motion, it is $\mu_0 - \mu_1 < 0$. If the outputs of a neuron in successive time intervals are independent, then their densities multiply, and so the log likelihood ratio after n neuronal evidence samples favoring upward motion becomes

$$\ln L_n = \frac{\mu_1 - \mu_0}{\sigma^2} \sum_{i=1}^{n} (x_i - y_i)$$

According to Gold and Shadlen (2001, 2007), this result suggests a biologically plausible implementation to solve the animal's decision problem: to accumulate the difference in spike rates over time of those neurons tuned to the upward direction vs. those tuned to the downward direction. If the motion stimulus shown has upward direction, this running total will on average increase per step; if the motion has downward direction, it will on average decrease. The absolute size of the average step depends on $\mu_1 - \mu_0$, the sharpness of the tuning of the neuronal populations involved, and also on the noise σ^2 in the biological system. Gold and Shadlen emphasize that the animal does not need to have any explicit knowledge about distributional parameters; essentially, it must keep track of, and contrast, the running activation total of two neuronal populations.

The expression for $\ln L_n$ clearly links these concepts to diffusion processes as a limit of many steps of variable size. Gold and Shadlen (2001, 2007) suggest that an animal tracks $\ln L_n$ until for the first time an upper or lower evidence threshold at $\pm a$ has been reached. In this view, the probability of a correct decision to a motion stimulus with upward (downward) direction corresponds to the probability to absorb at the upper (lower) barrier, and the decision time corresponds to the associated first-passage time. The drift of this diffusion process reflects the sharpness of the orientation tuning of the MT neurons; for example, the absolute value of $\mu_1 - \mu_0$ increases with motion strength. For large evidence thresholds a, decisions tend to be correct but slow, whereas for small a, decisions tend to be fast but error-prone. Gold and Shadlen (2001, 2007) suggest that animals choose an intermediate threshold value of a to settle this speed-accuracy trade-off by maximizing their temporal rate of reward.

The basic conceptual approach described above is part of a larger class of so-called sequential sampling models which have provided a dominant theoretical framework guiding computational and neurophysiological investigations of perceptual decision-making. Some recent applications, extensions, challenges, and alternatives to this approach are presented, for example, by O'Connell et al. (2018), Zylberberg et al. (2016), or Schall et al. (2011).

7.6.2 Random Walk Models of Discrimination and Choice Behavior in Animals

Random walk and diffusion models in animal studies have not only been used to describe mechanisms at the neuronal level but are also prominent in behavioral studies of discrimination and choice behavior. A characteristic example is the work of Blough (2011) on color discrimination in white carneaux pigeons. Traditionally, perceptual studies using animals have relied on analyzing the relative frequency of choice responses only. Blough (2011) argued that another relevant and informative variable is the time that animals take to arrive at their decisions. In his study, white carneaux pigeons discriminated color signals that increased in wavelength in eight steps from blue to green; the animals had to respond to the four signals with shorter (longer) wavelengths with a peck to a left (right) target spot. After considerable training, the birds learned to respond to the signals with the two shortest (most bluish) and the two longest (most greenish) wavelengths with an error rate below 5%; with the four intermediate wavelengths, the task remained difficult, and the choice proportions varied between 20 and 80%.

The frequency and latency of the responses to the eight color signals are shown as dots in Fig. 7.6. Clearly, as the color changes from blue to green, the proportion of right responses increases regularly. Also, the animals required more time the harder the discrimination was, with systematic changes in their response time distributions. For any given stimulus, correct responses were on average faster than incorrect responses.

Blough (2011) accounted for the response proportions and latency characteristics with a random walk model; it assumes that the animal accumulates noisy sensory evidence about the color of the signal in discrete time steps. As in Gold and Shadlen (2001, 2007) per step, this evidence is normally distributed, with a mean that depends on the wavelength of the stimulus, being positive (negative) for bluish (greenish) signals. A decision is made and the response executed when the accumulated evidence first reaches an upper or lower evidence threshold. An additional feature of his model is that across trials, the starting point and mean step size (i.e., the drift parameter) of the induced random walk are themselves normally distributed random variables. The lines in Fig. 7.6 show that the best fit of this model captures major characteristics of the frequency and latency data in considerable detail. Blough emphasizes that his model can help to disentangle the differential effects of response-reward and stimulus-reward associations, the former mainly affecting response frequency and the latter decision time. He concludes that the random walk model yields a plausible and coherent picture of the decision process underlying color discrimination in pigeons that is more complete than studies ignoring the latencies of the responses.

The argument of Blough (2011) to consider both the latency and the frequency of choice responses can be carried an important step further. Given that environmental signals and sensory systems are inherently noisy, adequate decisions and effective motor actions may require an animal to sample evidence over an extended period of time. For example, pollinators need to discriminate rewarding flowers from Batesian mimics; here, errors are typically cheap, and a quick but inaccurate strategy can be optimal. In other contexts, such as the avoidance of life-threatening predators, errors can be quite costly. Thus, most prey species take considerable time to scrutinize carefully their environment, especially when the predators are cryptic and actively hide or camouflage. These and many other situations have in common that there is a characteristic trade-off between speed and accuracy, so that animals must choose

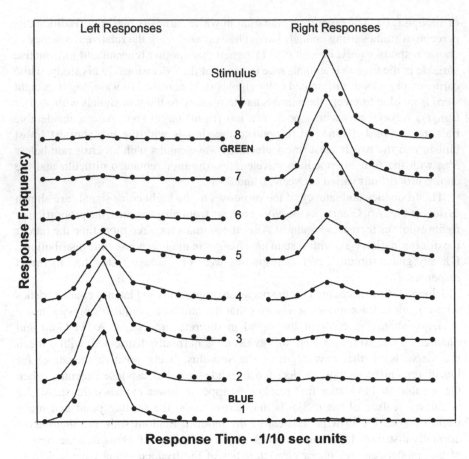

Fig. 7.6 Response frequency and latency of pigeons in a color discrimination experiment (after Blough 2011). The abscissa shows response time in steps 100 ms and the ordinate response frequency for each combination of color signal, the bird's response, and 100 ms latency time slot. The wavelength of the color signals increases from bottom (blue) to top (green). Bluish signals required left responses and greenish signals right responses

between fast-but-error-prone and accurate-but-slow strategies. Chittka et al. (2009) review characteristic patterns of speed-accuracy trade-offs in several biological contexts and explain the critical role of random walk and diffusion models to synthesize the observations in this context.

Chittka et al. (2003) provided ten bumblebees with eight virtual "flowers" whose locations changed from trial to trial. Four flowers were colored blue, and four had a greenish component; only the blue flowers contained a rewarding sucrose solution; the four others contained just water. Chittka et al. observed how often each bee landed on each color and measured their decision time, that is, the length of the flight time between flowers. The search strategies of individual bees differed considerably, and those bees taking more time were more accurate. Does this reflect

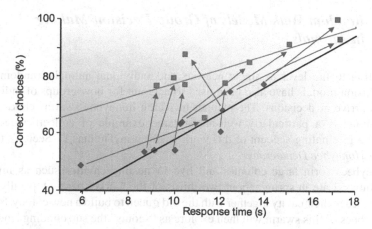

Fig. 7.7 Response times (abscissa) and proportion correct (ordinate) for ten bumblebees in a color discrimination task; the guessing level corresponds to 50% correct. Each pair of squares connected by an arrow shows the performance of a single bee when errors are cheap (lower left squares) vs. when they are costly (upper right squares). In nine of ten bees, costly errors reduce speed, and for all ten bees, they increase accuracy. From Chittka et al. (2003); with permission

a genuine speed-accuracy trade-off or simply individual variations of perceptual and motor limitations? In a second condition using the same bees, Chittka et al. offered an aversive quinine solution at the green distractor locations, making errors more costly. As shown in Fig. 7.7, under these conditions, nine of ten bees took more time to inspect each flower, and all ten bees improved their accuracy. Chittka et al. (2003) conclude that individual bees differ systematically in their relative preference for fast vs. accurate search strategies, but for nearly all of them, increasing the cost of errors will prolong decision time and reduce the error rate.

An important general conclusion drawn by Chittka et al. (2009) is that animals do not per se intend to excel at an (to them) arbitrary task posed by a human experimenter but optimize the relation of reward and effort. This is sometimes achieved by a fast and error-prone strategy, especially when errors are not too costly. Thus, joint analyses of response speed and accuracy are more informative and reduce ambiguity compared to analyses merely based on percentage correct. For a simple diffusion model underlying the account given by Chittka et al. (2009, Figure 2), see Exercise 2. More recently, Wang et al. (2015) and Ducatez et al. (2015) extended and generalized the findings of Chittka et al. (2003); they demonstrated speed-accuracy trade-offs and consistent individual speed vs. accuracy preferences in zebrafishes and Carib grackles. For a thorough review of related work, see, for example, Kacelnik et al. (2011) who characterize the random walk and diffusion framework aptly as "tug-of-war models" and contrast it with parallel race models; Pelé and Sueur (2013) and Abbott and Sherratt (2013) provide a detailed discussion of these and related models.

7.6.3 Random Walk Models of Group Decision-Making in Animals

In addition to the level of single neurons and individual animals, random walk and diffusion models have also been used to account for how groups of individual animals arrive at decisions. The manner in which honeybee swarms choose their future home is a particularly well-investigated example of collective decision-making; a fascinating account of this work is given in Thomas D. Seeley's (2010) book on *Honeybee Democracy*.

Honeybees form large colonies and live in nesting cavities such as hives or tree hollows. Late in spring, about two-thirds of the worker bees—typically some 10,000—leave their cavity together with the old queen to build a new colony. Several hundred bees of this swarm will then explore as "scouts" the surrounding landscape for potential cavities, locate and inspect several possibilities, and select a favorite for their new domicile. Choosing the right place to live is a decision of vital importance because the new colony will only survive if its new hive provides sufficient space, warmth, and protection. This decision is therefore made not by a few individual bees but by several hundred bees acting collectively, and their collective choice almost always favors the site that best satisfies the multiple criteria of an ideal nesting cavity. It is this most remarkable process of collective decision-making that Seeley refers to as "honeybee democracy".

Karl von Frisch discovered that bees indicate features of attractive sites to their fellows by complex forms of movement—the "bee dance", as von Frisch named it, is the language in which bees communicate. This form of communication is also used when it comes to selecting a new hive. Scout bees collect information for several hours or even several days. They come and go from the swarm and indicate their commitment to a site by dances that are graded in strength, thereby stimulating as yet uncommitted scouts to visit the favored site. Thus, there is much moment-to-moment variation in the strength of the signals activating additional scouts to visit any given site. The better the site, the more scouts will dance for it, and the more additional scouts are attracted to it which means that the evidence supporting a particular location tends to accumulate most rapidly at the best site. A scout "votes" for a site by spending time at it, with the number of scouts rising faster at better sites.

The swarm ultimately reaches a decision based on a quorum, that is, on a sufficient number of scouts at one of the nest sites rather than by reaching full consensus among all dancing scouts. According to Seeley, unlike consensus-sensing, quorum-sensing enables fast, yet accurate, decisions and optimizes the speed-accuracy trade-off. The bees monitor the scouts at each site, and once the quorum has been reached, the swarm moves to the new hive.

As illustrated in Fig. 7.8, in the case of a swarm choosing between two possible nest sites, the evidence provided by any scout for one alternative can be seen as evidence against the other site, so in effect the evidence can be represented and accumulated as a single differential total. As scouts explore the environment, the

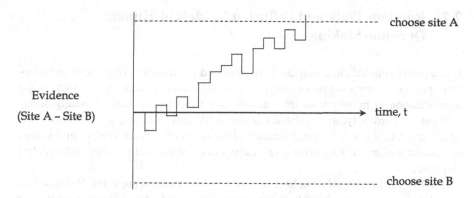

Fig. 7.8 Seeley's (2010) random walk model of bees choosing a hive site. The evidence about two potential hive sites is accumulated over time (abscissa) as a single total (ordinate). Evidence for site A increases the total, while evidence for site B decreases it. A choice is made when the net gain in evidence for one site exceeds a threshold level, the so-called quorum (after Seeley 2010)

swarm acquires more evidence regarding the two alternatives, and at any one time, only one site will have accumulated a nonzero level of evidence in its favor. In the words of Thomas Seeley (2010, ch. 9), "the accumulation of evidence can be thought of as a random walk along a time line where the positive direction represents increasing evidence for one of the alternatives and the negative direction represents increasing evidence for the other alternative (Fig. 7.8). The drift of the evidence line up or down denotes the tendency of the line to move toward the better alternative, and the jaggedness of the line represents the noisiness or uncertainty in the incoming evidence. It turns out that this random walk or diffusion model of decision making implements the statistically optimal" procedure.

Seeley (2010) summarizes in great detail the evidence supporting his conceptualization of the bee's collective choice of a new hive, shown in Fig. 7.8. It seems quite remarkable that the same conceptual framework developed to understand decision-making in primate brains (cf., Sect. 7.6.1) also helps to account for the dynamics of the collective decision-making process in honeybee swarms. Perhaps even more remarkable, very similar evidence accumulation and quorum-sensing mechanisms capture in considerable detail the dynamics of collective decisions reached, for example, by ant colonies (*Temnothorax albipennis*) which reliably select the best of several potential nest sites (Pratt 2005). Seeley (2010) argues that the striking convergence in the design of decision-making systems built of neurons, bees, and ants reflects independent evolutions of a general diffusion-based scheme of implementing robust, efficient, and often nearly optimal decision-making. Detailed descriptions and extensions of random walk and diffusion models of collective decision-making in animals appear, for example, in Passino and Seeley (2006), Pratt (2005), Seeley et al. (2006), or Wolf et al. (2013).

7.7   Random Walk and Diffusion Models of Human Decision-Making

It is a priori plausible that humans have inherited from their evolutionary ancestors time-proven information processing and decision-making mechanisms, such as the accumulation of noisy partial information over time or thresholding and quorum-sensing. Accordingly, most related random walk and diffusion applications refer, specifically, to the way in which humans make decisions. The literature in this area is vast, so we can only mention a few exemplary studies and point to some central references.

Highly relevant signals that have to compete for attention are often designed in a correlated, redundant fashion, both in naturalistic and in technical environments. For example, ambulances toot horns and flash lights to warn off other traffic. Underlying these composite displays is the idea that redundant signals will perhaps be more conspicuous, that is, be detected more easily or earlier, than either of these signals alone. Coactivation models (Miller 1982) of information processing assume that sensory activations induced by the individual signals combine and thus will on average reach an activation threshold earlier than the activation induced by each signal individually.

Diffusion models such as the Wiener process have helped to make this general notion more specific and to compare it to quantitative data (Schwarz 1994). For a single signal, they assume that noisy partial information is continuously accumulated until an evidence barrier is reached for the first time. With redundant signals, such as a tone and a visual stimulus, the separate stochastic activation processes are superimposed within a more central processing stage onto which both afferent pathways converge. To test this idea, an experimental standard paradigm is to manipulate the temporal offset τ between the two signals.

With the onset of the first signal, sensory information about it starts to be accumulated. If the temporal offset τ of the signals is sufficiently long, this process alone will often reach the threshold and trigger the motor response, even before the trailing signal is presented. Alternatively, especially with short temporal offsets, the barrier will often not yet have been reached when the second signal is presented, and then the two accumulation processes superimpose and therefore form a diffusion process defined by

$$X_{R,\tau}(t) = X_1(t) + X_2(t - \tau) \qquad \text{where } t, \tau \geq 0$$

This superimposed accumulation processes $X_{R,\tau}(t)$ will on average reach a given detection threshold earlier than each of the constituent accumulation processes individually.

Figure 7.9 shows the fit of this simple model to data of a detailed study by Miller (1986) in which observers responded as soon as possible to a visual or an auditory signal, whichever was detected first. The left (right) part of Fig. 7.9 refers to trials when the auditory (visual) signal was presented first, by a head start indicated on

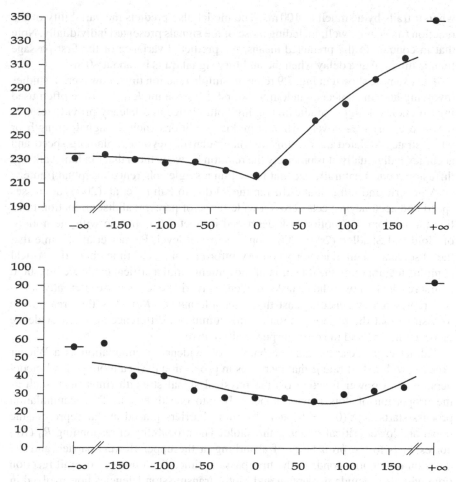

Fig. 7.9 Fit of a superposition diffusion model to the reaction time data of Miller (1986). Human observers responded as soon as possible to a visual or an auditory signal, whichever was detected first. The temporal head start of the visual signal is indicated on the abscissa; negative values refer to trials in which the auditory signal was presented first. The left-most and right-most data points refer to trials in which the auditory or the visual signal, respectively, was presented alone. The upper panel refers to the means (ordinate) and the lower panel to the standard deviations (ordinate) of the reaction times; the lines show the prediction of the superposition diffusion model. After Schwarz (1994)

the abscissa. The left-most and right-most data points refer to trials in which the auditory or the visual signal, respectively, was presented alone. As can be seen in the upper panel, responses to the auditory signal alone were on average quite a bit faster (231 ms) than responses to the visual signal alone (348 ms); they were also clearly less variable (lower panel). The superposition model captures many aspects of the data in considerable quantitative detail: responses are fastest when both signals are presented simultaneously, and the faster auditory signal speeds up responses even when it trails by as much as 100 ms. The model also predicts the variability of the reaction times quite well, including those of the signals presented individually. Note that in contrast to the predicted means, the predicted variance of the first-passage time is minimal at a delay when the auditory signal trails by about 80 ms.

The example shown in Fig. 7.9 refers to simple reaction time; however, in studies involving human subjects, random walk and diffusion models are more often used in two-choice designs. Studies involving both choice and latency provide tests of how these variables covary when stimulus conditions such as signal strength or when strategy-related instructions are manipulated. Beyond explaining speed and accuracy individually, it is precisely the relation between them that random walk and diffusion models naturally account for within a single coherent conceptual frame.

A generic and influential diffusion model due to Palmer et al. (2005) addresses speed and accuracy aspects across a wide range of perceptual discrimination tasks like the random dot motion task described in Sect. 7.6.1. In line with the notions of Gold and Shadlen (2001, 2007) on a neuronal level, Palmer et al. assume that the observers accumulate noisy sensory information across time about the critical stimulus feature (e.g., the direction of movement) until a critical evidence threshold is first reached. In two-choice tasks, evidence favoring one response alternative (say, R_a) represents evidence against the other alternative (R_b); it is thus reasonable to assume that the observers monitor the cumulated difference between evidence favoring the one and the other response alternative.

Palmer et al. describe this mechanism of evidence accumulation as a Wiener process, with a drift rate μ that increases in proportion to (in a more general model version, as a power function of) the physical signal strength (intensity), such as the proportion of dots moving coherently into one direction. The accumulation process starts at $X(0) = 0$, and absorbing barriers placed at $\pm a$ represent the upper and lower critical evidence threshold. The probability of responding R_a (R_b) corresponds to the probability of absorbing at the upper (lower) barrier, and the decision time corresponds to the first-passage time. The observed overall reaction time will also include perceptual and motor transmission latencies not involved in the decision process, and the mean of these lumped "residual" latencies is denoted by t_R. Note that in behavioral studies, only the ultimate overt choice and its latency are observable, not the accumulation process itself. Therefore, the spatial scale of the diffusion process is arbitrary, and Palmer et al. use the normalization $\sigma^2 = 1$. Explicit accuracy and reaction time predictions are considered in Exercise 2.

Using a representative variety of perceptual tasks, Palmer et al. (2005) applied this model to speed and accuracy data of trained human observers. The authors describe efficient procedures to estimate the parameters of the model and conclude that it accounts for major findings, such as varying the stimulus strength, response modalities, the nature of the task, or critical properties of the stimuli. Figure 7.10 shows data from a direction discrimination task involving dynamic random dot fields. Naturally, in discrimination tasks involving arrays of randomly moving dots, accuracy tends to be higher with increasing viewing time. In three separate speed conditions, two observers were instructed to stop inspecting the motion fields such that in the most difficult condition (lowest coherence), they would respond after

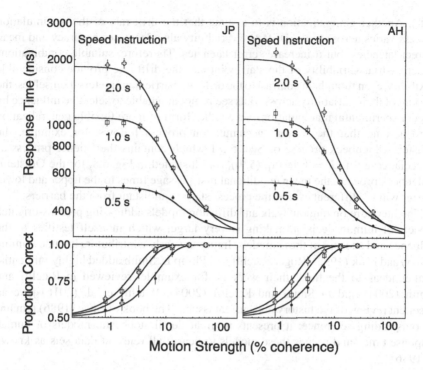

Fig. 7.10 Fit of the Palmer et al. (2005) diffusion model to the accuracy (ordinate, lower panel) and reaction time (ordinate, upper panel) data of two observers in a direction discrimination task with dynamic random dot fields. The abscissa refers to the motion coherence of the random dots; measurements were taken at seven coherence levels. In three separate speed instruction conditions, the targeted response time in the most difficult condition (lowest coherence) was 500, 1000, or 2000 ms. Note the logarithmic scale of the abscissa and the ordinate of the upper panel. After Palmer et al. (2005)

about 500, 1000, or 2000 ms; motion coherence was varied in logarithmic steps from 0.8% to 51.2%. Figure 7.10 shows that the Palmer et al. model provides an excellent quantitative fit both to the accuracy data and to the mean reaction times at all motion coherence levels and under all three speed conditions.

A major limitation of the model is that the conditional mean first-passage time is the same for absorbing at the upper and lower barrier (cf., Exercises 6 and 7 of Chap. 4). It thus predicts equal mean reaction times for correct and error responses. Empirically, errors are often slower than correct responses when the task is difficult (as in the Palmer et al. study), and they tend to be faster than correct responses for easy tasks.

Palmer et al. discuss several possible generalizations of their diffusion model to overcome this limitation. One generalization is to assume that the starting point of the accumulation process varies across trials. Start point variability decreases accuracy and both conditional mean first-passage times, but it reduces error latencies more than correct latencies (i.e., absorptions at the barrier in the direction of the drift). Another generalization is to assume that the drift rate of the accumulation process varies across trials. Drift rate variability also decreases accuracy and mean correct latencies, but it increases error latencies. Therefore, suitable combinations of across-trial variability of the start point and the drift rate provide considerable flexibility, even though, in contrast to the drift and barrier parameters themselves, the amount of their variability across trials seems not amenable to selective influence by direct experimental manipulation. Yet another form of more flexible generalization is to assume that the sensory accumulation process follows, for example, the Ornstein-Uhlenbeck process of Sect. 5.3.1 which contains the Wiener process as a special case (cf., $k = 0$ in Eq. (5.9)). As illustrated in Fig. 6.8, for the Ornstein-Uhlenbeck process, the mean conditional first-passage times to the upper and lower barrier will be different even if the process starts equidistant from the barriers.

The literature on random walk and diffusion models addressing process-oriented aspects of human decision-making is very large, which in itself testifies to the influence and success of these models. Important early contributors include Laming (1968) and Link (1992). Roger Ratcliff and Philip L. Smith added highly influential further ideas to the field; their work is, for example, reviewed in Ratcliff and Smith (2004) and in Smith and Ratcliff (2004); Ratcliff et al. (2016) give an excellent review of the history and current issues. The book of Luce (1986) remains an outstanding reference; it presents in great detail stochastic models of human response times and relates these models to nearly all relevant data sets as known of 1986.

7.8 Some Further Applications of Random Walk and Diffusion Models in the Behavioral and Life Sciences

We conclude this section by briefly noting a few original or less common applications of random walk and diffusion models in areas not covered in the previous sections.

Marma and Deutsch (1973) use a simple random walk representation as a general model of conflict between opponents of unequal resources and capabilities. In their scenario, two conflicting parties compete in successive direct encounters for a single scarce commodity, such as votes, territory, or market share. Marma and Deutsch identify three major components governing such conflicts: (1) the relative proportion of total resources initially available to each party (e.g., rich or powerful parties vs. underdogs), (2) the ability to win any single encounter (e.g., more skill or higher popularity) (3) the proportion of the total resources which are at risk in each single encounter (e.g., bold, big-risk battles vs. cautious skirmishes).

Translated into the scenario of random walks starting at x between absorbing barriers at 0 and a, and with single step probability p, these components correspond to the quantities x/a, p, and $1/a$, respectively. Analyzing the way in which these different factors influence the winning probability (Sect. 2.3.2), Marma and Deutsch derive several general strategic conclusions. For moderate advantages of initial resources ($x \approx a/2$), and for moderate or small proportions of the total resources at risk in each encounter (i.e., when a is large), small changes in p are much more important than the initial relative resources. Parties with large x/a but small p should aim at high-risk contests because protracted small-scale encounters with adversive odds will wear them down. Parties with a small proportion of initial resources x/a (underdogs) but larger p are better off to avoid big risks and should prefer small-scale encounters (guerilla warfare tactics). For nearly even contests (when $p \approx \frac{1}{2}$), increasing x or $a - x$ (e.g., raising the war effort by mass mobilization) will lead to long-drawn contests of attrition.

A related random walk model of bargaining and warfare has been presented by Smith and Stam (2004). These authors investigate the critical role of prior beliefs about p and discuss conditions under which a negotiated settlement is acceptable for both parties.

Yasuda (1975) proposed a diffusion model to explain matrimonial distances in humans, that is, the spatial distance between the birthplaces of mates. His account is based on similar assumptions as the model of Broadbent and Kendall (1953), described in Sect. 7.4. He assumes that a person may in any given short time interval come across a critical event (e.g., find a partner) with probability density $g(t)$ and then stop moving around. Yasuda assumes that the stopping time has a gamma density g and then derives the distribution of the radial distance an individual will move till the moment of the stopping time. He successfully fits this model to matrimonial distances in Japan and Italy and accounts for some qualitative differences between urban and rural populations.

Castellano and Cermelli (2011) use a random walk framework to model the way in which females (e.g., gray tree frogs) choose mates. In their account, a female choosing a mate successively evaluates the attractiveness (quality, q_i) of all available male candidates $i = 1, \ldots, n$. Among males, the quality (fitness) q has some distribution, and the aim of the female is to maximize the expected q-value of the male ultimately chosen. However, the assessment of any male's quality is necessarily noisy, imperfect, and indirect, as it is based on phenotypic signals that covary with, but are not equal to, q_i. Each evaluation of a male candidate by the female results in a binary 1/0 verdict. After all n candidates have been screened, a new evaluation round starts in the same manner, to increase the reliability of the female's choice. For each male individually, the 1/0 verdicts are accumulated as in a random walk that in each round either stays put or moves ahead one step. The female will choose the first male reaching an acceptance threshold, corresponding to the "choosiness" of the female. The model provides a coherent framework to investigate different mechanisms and strategies of mating decisions. For example, it predicts that under time pressure, females will trade the accuracy of population sampling (the number n of males sampled) against a more reliable assessment of each individual (the time spent for evaluating each mate).

Helland and Raviv (2008) use a random walk model to discuss the optimal jury size in trials in which a unanimous verdict of conviction or acquittal must be reached. Their model assumes that each of n jurors initially evaluates the evidence presented in court; this evaluation corresponds with probability u to the true state of nature (i.e., the defendant is guilty vs. innocent). In their model, the outcome of this initial evaluation forms the starting state of a random walk as defined by the number of jurors currently supporting conviction. In subsequent rounds of deliberation, each juror changes or maintains his or her current verdict with equal probability of $\frac{1}{2}$. This stage therefore forms a symmetric random walk, as discussed in Sect. 2.1. The final verdict is reached when all jurors support conviction (absorbing state n) or when all jurors support acquittal (absorbing state 0). Helland and Raviv demonstrate that in their model the probability of a jury committing an error (of either type) is independent of the number n of jurors and is equal to the probability $1 - u$ that a single juror would commit an error. They conclude that the optimal jury size is $n = 1$: reducing the number n of jurors used in a trial, the cost of conducting a trial is reduced without increasing the probability of committing errors. Curley et al. (2019) provide a comprehensive review of recent random walk and diffusion accounts of juror decision-making in a legal context.

7.9 Exercises

1. To derive the expected squared displacement after $n = 2$ steps in the model of Fig. 7.3, let us assume that both steps have unit length and denote for simplicity the first two turning angles as α and β. Then the position (x, y) of the walk after two steps is given by $x = \cos(\alpha) + \cos(\alpha + \beta)$ and $y = \sin(\alpha) + \sin(\alpha + \beta)$. Clearly, the squared displacement is $x^2 + y^2$, which we write in the form of $(x + iy)(x - iy)$. Thus,

$$x + iy = \cos(\alpha) + \cos(\alpha + \beta) + i[\sin(\alpha) + \sin(\alpha + \beta)]$$

$$= \cos(\alpha) + i\sin(\alpha) + \cos(\alpha + \beta) + i\sin(\alpha + \beta)$$

$$= \exp(i\alpha) + \exp[i(\alpha + \beta)]$$

by Euler's identity. In a similar way, we have

$$x - iy = \exp(-i\alpha) + \exp[-i(\alpha + \beta)]$$

Multiplying $(x + iy)(x - iy)$ out, we get

$$x^2 + y^2 = 2 + \exp(i\beta) + \exp(-i\beta)$$

$$= 2 + \cos(\beta) + i\sin(\beta) + \cos(\beta) - i\sin(\beta)$$

$$= 2 + 2\cos(\beta)$$

Therefore, the expected squared displacement after the first two steps will be $E[\mathbf{R}_2^2] = 2 + 2E[\cos(\beta)]$, where the expected cosine of the turning angle depends on the density of this angle. For example, when this density is sharply concentrated around zero, then the expected squared displacement after two steps will be close to 4, as the walk proceeds simply along the abscissa, toward $(2, 0)$. In contrast, when the density is sharply concentrated at π (180°), then the two steps will tend to be back and forth. In this case, $\mathsf{E}[\cos(\beta)] \approx -1$, and $\mathsf{E}[\mathbf{R}_2^2]$ will be close to zero.

Explain why under the assumptions made, $\mathsf{E}[\mathbf{R}_2^2]$ is independent of the angle α. Generalize this scheme first to $n = 3$ and then to general n. To this end, first assume that $\mathsf{E}[\sin(\beta)] = 0$ which means that the movement is not tortuous and on average the animal "homes in". Argue that the expected step length $\mathbf{L}$ enters only as a factor, as long as $\mathbf{L}$ and the turning angle are independent.

2. Many studies looking at the speed-accuracy trade-off in animal cognition use experimental designs in which the animal must choose between two response alternatives; in these situations, the chance level of responding is often 50% correct (Fig. 7.7). A basic model (e.g., Chittka et al. 2009, Figure 2) generating a speed-accuracy trade-off function assumes that the animal accumulates noisy sensory evidence across time until for the first time, an evidence threshold supporting the one or the other response is reached. This accumulation process is often conceptualized as a Wiener process between two absorbing barriers at $\pm a$ that starts at zero. The drift rate of the process depends on the actual stimulus presented and is positive (negative) for stimuli for which the upper (lower) barrier is correct. Consider a stimulus for which the upper barrier is the correct response, so that $\mu > 0$.

According to this simple diffusion model, the probability $x(a)$ of a correct response is the probability to absorb at the upper barrier (cf., Eq. (4.44))

$$x(a) = \frac{1}{1 + \exp\left(-\frac{2a\mu}{\sigma^2}\right)}$$

and the mean decision time $y(a)$ is the mean first-passage time (cf., Exercise 6 in Chap. 4)

$$y(a) = \frac{a}{\mu} \cdot \frac{1 - \exp\left(-\frac{2a\mu}{\sigma^2}\right)}{1 + \exp\left(-\frac{2a\mu}{\sigma^2}\right)}$$

The animal governs the strategic speed-accuracy trade-off by choosing the threshold evidence parameter a.

Solve $x(a)$ for a, and insert into $y(a)$ to obtain the explicit form of the implied speed-accuracy trade-off function $f : x \to y = f(x)$ for $\frac{1}{2} \le x < 1$. Investigate the nature of f, and relate its features to Chittka et al.'s (2009) conclusion that animals have no interest per se in excelling at tasks in which only accuracy is measured and that sometimes "good enough is best".

3. Assume that the reward of a correct choice is $r > 0$ and the cost of an error is $c \geq 0$. For a given accuracy x, the animal will on average make $1/f(x)$ choices per time unit, with f given by the previous Exercise 2. How should the accuracy level x (via adjusting the evidence threshold, a) be chosen so as to maximize the overall rate of gain? Explain the dependency of this maximum on r, c, μ, and σ, and relate this to the findings of Chittka et al. (2003) shown in Fig. 7.7.

4. A concept of the speed-accuracy trade-off not based on the variation of the evidence barriers is known as the conditional accuracy function (CAF; e.g., Luce 1986). Assume as in Exercise 2 that the animal accumulates noisy sensory evidence as in a Wiener process until for the first time, a threshold at a or $-b$ supporting the one or the other response is reached. Assume that the drift μ is positive and that absorbing at a (at $-b$) produces the correct (incorrect) response. Across many trials, it is then possible to look at the relative proportion of correct responses for successive (short) bins of decision (i.e., first-passage) times (cf., Figs. 4.8 and 4.9). This type of analysis traces, for a given pair of barriers, the time course of response accuracy as the latency of the decisions varies. Use Eqs. (4.64) and (4.65) and the relation Eq. (4.66) to express for the Wiener process the theoretical CAF, that is, the conditional probability that the absorption occurs at a, given the first-passage time equals t. Plot this CAF for $0 < t < 300$ using the parameters in the figures cited.

5. If in the superposition model underlying Fig. 7.9 the drift and variance of $X_i(t)$ are μ_i, σ_i^2, and their correlation is ϱ, then derive the mean and variance of the first-passage time to a threshold a when either signal is presented alone and when both signals are presented simultaneously (cf., Exercise 4 of Chap. 4).

6. As shown in Fig. 7.9, the diffusion superposition model predicts that the variance of the first-passage time of the superimposed diffusion process $\{X_{R,\tau}(t)\}$ is minimal when the delay of the auditory signal is about 80 ms (for the specific parameters underlying this figure). Explain this prediction qualitatively by considering the behavior of the model when the accumulation process induced by the signal presented first has zero variance.

7. Assume that across independent trials (realizations), the drift of an induced Wiener diffusion process is itself a normally distributed random variable μ, with mean u and variance η^2. Use conditional expectation and conditional variance (e.g., Eq. (2.54)) to show that

$$\mathsf{E}[X(t)] = ut \qquad \text{and also} \qquad \mathsf{Var}[X(t)] = \sigma^2 t + \eta^2 t^2$$

Explain why the latter result implies that the unconditional process is not a Wiener process again.

The results for $\mathsf{E}[X(t)]$ and $\mathsf{Var}[X(t)]$ mean that if one registered at a fixed time t the position $X(t)$ of many independent realizations of this randomized diffusion process, $X(t)$ would be normally distributed, with mean ut and variance $\sigma^2 t + \eta^2 t^2$. However, the diffusion coefficient *within* any of these realizations (e.g., the variance of the displacement per time unit) would still only be σ^2.

Consider the limiting "ballistic" case of $\sigma = 0$, and explain why in this case the probability to absorb at the upper barrier is $\Phi(u/\eta)$, independent of the numerical barrier values, a and $-b$.

8. The covariance of a diffusion process at times t and $t + \tau$ is (cf. Sect. 5.3.2)

$$\text{cov}[X(t), X(t + \tau)] = \text{cov}\{X(t), X(t) + [X(t + \tau) - X(t)]\}$$

$$= \text{cov}[X(t), X(t)] + \text{cov}[X(t), X(t + \tau) - X(t)]$$

For any process with independent increments, the second cov−Term is zero, as it refers to the non-overlapping time intervals $[0, t]$ and $[t, t + \tau]$. For the Wiener process, the first term is $\text{Var}[X(t)] = \sigma^2 t$.

Show that the corresponding result for the randomized diffusion process considered in the previous Exercise 7 is

$$\text{cov}[X(t), X(t + \tau)] = \sigma^2 t + \eta^2 t(t + \tau)$$

Explain why in the randomized diffusion process, the increments $X(t)$ and $X(t + \tau) - X(t)$ are not independent even though they refer to non-overlapping time intervals.

9. Explain why in a Wiener process (all other things being equal), additional across-trial variability of the start point or the drift rate generally reduces the accuracy. For example, use Eq. (6.26) with $\mu > 0$ to compute the accuracy $\pi_+(x)$ for a Wiener process with absorbing barriers at 0 and a always starting at $0 < x < a$. Compare this with the accuracy $p\pi_+(x+\Delta)+(1-p)\pi_+(x-\Delta)$ in a randomized version in which the start is with probability p at $x+\Delta$ and with probability $1-p$ at $x - \Delta$. Note that $\pi_+(x)$ is a concave function, so that the line segment between any two points on $\pi_+(x)$ lies below the function.

References

The mathematical literature on random walk and diffusion models is vast; it differs widely in the coverage of applied aspects and in the level of mathematical rigor. Thus, a few comments on some of the titles listed below may be helpful as a first orientation. In addition to all sources cited in the text, I have added a number of further references which seemed to me particularly helpful at the level addressed in this book.

Ross (2019) is an excellent introduction to probability models; his (1996) book as well as Grimmett and Stirzaker (2001) provides an elegant, modern mathematical treatment of the topics covered in Chaps. 2–6 at a more advanced formal level. The detailed and concise treatment of stochastic processes by Cox and Miller (1965) resonates very well with the needs of applied modeling work in the life sciences, where the book remains hugely prominent. Feller's (1968, 1971) two volumes are a classic and ingenious introduction to probability theory, including random walk (in vol. I) and diffusion theory (in vol. II). The thorough two-volume course by Karlin and Taylor (1975, 1981) combines mathematical rigor with a number of interesting applications to the life sciences. The stimulating book of Berg (1993) reviews conceptual random walk ideas in biology. A modern guide to first-passage processes, focusing mainly on a physical context, is Redner (2001). The books of Borodin and Salminen (2015) and of Karatzas and Shreve (1998) present the mathematical basis of diffusion theory at a rigorous, advanced technical level.

Some of the classical articles and books provide superb, crystal-clear analyses and have remained remarkably readable even today; they are highly recommended. Among them are the independent and simultaneous original derivation of the first-passage time distribution Eq. 4.22 by Erwin Schrödinger (1915) and Marian von Smoluchowski (1915), the Kohlrausch and Schrödinger (1926) derivation of the Ornstein-Uhlenbeck process from the Ehrenfest urn model, Fürth's (1920) original work on correlated random walks, and the masterful treatment of Darling and Siegert (1953). An English translation of von Smoluchowski's work can be found

© Springer Nature Switzerland AG 2022
W. Schwarz, *Random Walk and Diffusion Models*,
https://doi.org/10.1007/978-3-031-12100-5

in Chandrasekhar et al. (2000); for a collection of Schrödinger's work, see his *Collected Papers*, vol. 1.

Stewart's (2012) book is a masterful exposition of most of the mathematical tools used in this book; more advanced topics are systematically presented in Wylie and Barrett (1995). Stewart and Day (2016) provide an excellent text to explain how calculus and probability relate to biology, with a style that maintains rigor without being overly formal.

I. Books

AALEN, O O., BORGAN, O. AND GJESSING, H.K. (2008). *Survival and Event History Analysis: A Process Point View*. Springer, New York.

ABRAMOWITZ, M. AND STEGUN, I.A. (1965). *Handbook of Mathematical Functions*. Dover, New York.

AGRESTI, A. (2013). *Categorical Data Analysis*, 3rd ed. Wiley, New York.

BERG, H.C. (1993) *Random Walks in Biology*, expanded ed. Princeton University Press, Princeton.

BHARUCHA-REID, A.T. (1997). *Elements of the Theory of Markov Processes and Their Applications*. Dover, Mineola.

BORODIN, A. AND SALMINEN, P. (2015). *Handbook of Brownian Motion – Facts and Formulae* (corr. 3rd printing). Birkhäuser, Basel.

BULMER, M.G. (2003). *Francis Galton: Pioneer of Heredity and Biometry*. Johns Hopkins University Press, Baltimore.

CHANDRASEKHAR, S., KAC, M. AND SMOLUCHOWSKI, R. (2000), *Marian Smoluchowski: His Life and Scientific Work*. Polish Scientific Publishers PWN, Warszawa.

COX, D.R. AND MILLER, H.D. (1965). *The Theory of Stochastic Processes*. Chapman and Hall, London.

CROW, J.F. AND KIMURA, M. (1970). *An Introduction to Population Genetics Theory*. Harper and Row, New York.

FELLER, W. (1968, 1971). *An Introduction to Probability Theory and its Applications*. Vol. I, 3rd ed.; Vol. II, 2nd ed. Wiley, New York.

GOEL, N.S. AND RICHTER-DYN, N. (1974). *Stochastic Models in Biology*. Academic Press, New York.

GOULD, S.J. (1996). *Full House. The Spread of Excellence from Plato to Darwin*. Harmony Books, New York.

GREGORY, R.L. (2015). *Eye and Brain: The Psychology of Seeing*, 5th ed. Princeton University Press, Princeton.

GRIMMETT, G.R., AND STIRZAKER, D.R. (2001). *Probability and Random Processes. Problems and Solutions*, 3rd ed. Oxford University Press, Oxford.

KEMENY, J.G., AND SNELL, J.L. (1983). *Finite Markov Chains*. Springer, New York.

JACOBS, M.H. (1967) *Diffusion Processes*. Springer, Berlin.

KARATZAS, I. AND SHREVE, S.E. (1998). *Brownian Motion and Stochastic Calculus*, 2nd ed. Springer, New York.

KARLIN, S. AND TAYLOR, H.M. (1975) *A First Course in Stochastic Processes* (2nd ed.). Academic Press, San Diego.

© Springer Nature Switzerland AG 2022
W. Schwarz, *Random Walk and Diffusion Models*,
https://doi.org/10.1007/978-3-031-12100-5

KARLIN, S. AND TAYLOR, H.M. (1981) *A Second Course in Stochastic Processes*. Academic Press, New York.

LAMING, D.R.J. (1968). *Information Theory of Choice Reaction Time*. Wiley, New York.

LEFEBVRE, M. (2007). *Applied Stochastic Processes*. Springer, New York.

LEWIS, M.A., MAINI, P.K., AND PETROVSKII, S.V. (EDS.) (2013). *Dispersal, Individual Movement and Spatial Ecology. A Mathematical Perspective*. Springer, Berlin and Heidelberg.

LINK, S.W. (1992). *The Wave Theory of Difference and Similarity*. Lawrence Erlbaum, Hillsdale.

LUCE, R.D. (1986). *Response Times: Their Role in Inferring Elementary Mental Organization*. Oxford University Press, Oxford.

OKUBO, A. (1980). *Diffusion and Ecological Problems: Mathematical Models*. Springer, Berlin.

OKUBO, A. AND LEVIN, S.A. (2010). *Diffusion and Ecological Problems. Modern Perspectives*, 2nd ed. Springer, Berlin.

REDNER, S. (2001). *A Guide to First-Passage Processes*. Cambridge University Press, Cambridge.

ROSS, S.M. (2019). *Introduction to Probability Models*, 12th ed. Academic Press, San Diego.

ROSS, S.M. (1996). *Stochastic Processes*, 2nd ed. Academic Press, London.

SCHRÖDINGER, E. (1984). *Collected Papers. Vol. I: Contributions to Statistical Mechanics*. Vieweg, Braunschweig.

SEELEY, T.D. (2010). *Honeybee Democracy*. Princeton University Press, Princeton.

SMITH, G.D. (1985). *Numerical Solution of Partial Differential Equations. Finite Difference Methods*. Third Edition (corrected 2004). Oxford University Press, Oxford.

SMOLUCHOWSKI, M. VON (1923). *Abhandlungen über die Brownsche Bewegung und verwandte Erscheinungen. [Essays on Brownian Movement and Similar Phenomena]*. Ed. R. Fürth. Ostwalds Klassiker, vol. 207. Akademische Verlagsgesellschaft, Leipzig.

STEWART, J. (2012). *Calculus*. (7th ed.) Brooks/Cole, Belmont.

STEWART, J. AND DAY, T. (2016) *Biocalculus. Calculus for the Life Sciences*. Cengage, Boston.

TUCKWELL, H.C. (1995). *Elementary Applications of Probability Theory*, 2nd ed. Chapman and Hall/CRC, Boca Raton.

TURCHIN, P. (1998) *Quantitative Analysis of Movement: Measuring and Modeling Population Redistribution of Plants and Animals*. Sinauer, Sunderland.

WYLIE, C.R. AND BARRETT, L.C. (1995) *Advanced Engineering Mathematics* (6th ed.). McGraw-Hill, New York.

II. Articles

ABBOTT, K.R. AND SHERRATT, T.N. (2013). *Optimal sampling and signal detection: Unifying models of attention and speed-accuracy trade-offs. Behavioral Ecology*, **24**, 605–616.

BALKA J.D., ANTHONY F. AND MCNICHOLAS, P. D. (2009). *Review and implementation of cure models based on first hitting times for Wiener processes. Lifetime Data Analysis*, **15**, 147–176.

BERGER, J. AND POPE, D. (2011). *Can losing lead to winning? Management Science*, **57**, 817–827.

BERGMAN, C.M., SCHAEFER, J.A. AND LUTTICH, S.N. (2000) *Caribou movement as a correlated random walk. Oecologia*, **123**, 364–374.

BLOUGH, D.S. (2011). *A random-walk model of accuracy and reaction time applied to three experiments on pigeon visual discrimination. Journal of Experimental Psychology: Animal Behavior Processes*, **37**, 133–150.

BROADBENT, S.R. AND KENDALL, D.G. (1953) *The random walk of Trichostrongylus Retortaeformis. Biometrics*, **9**, 460–466.

CASTELLANO, S. AND CERMELLI, P. (2011). *Sampling and assessment accuracy in mate choice: A random-walk model of information processing in mating decision. Journal of Theoretical Biology*, **274**, 161–169.

CHEN, T. AND FAN, Q. (2018). *A functional data approach to model score difference process in professional basketball games. Journal of Applied Statistics*, **45**, 112–127.

CHITTKA, L., DYER, A.G., BOCK, F. AND DORNHAUS, A. (2003). *Bees trade off foraging speed for accuracy. Nature*, **424**, 388.

CHITTKA, L., SKORUPSKI, P. AND RAINE, N.E. (2009). *Speed-accuracy tradeoffs in animal decision making. Trends in Ecology and Evolution*, **24**, 400–407.

CODLING, E.A., PLANK, M.J. AND BENHAMOU, S. (2008). *Random walk models in biology. Journal of the Royal Society Interface*, **5**, 813–834.

CURLEY, L.J., MACLEAN, R., MURRAY, J., POLLOCK, A.C. AND LAYBOURN, P. (2019). *Threshold point utilisation in juror decision-making, Psychiatry, Psychology and Law*, **26**, 110–128.

DARLING, D.A. AND SIEGERT, A.J.F. (1953). *The first passage problem for a continuous Markov process. The Annals of Mathematical Statistics*, **24**, 624–639.

DUCATEZ, S., AUDET, J.N. AND LEFEBVRE, L. (2015). *Problem-solving and learning in Carib grackles: individuals show a consistent speed-accuracy trade-off. Animal Cognition*, **18**, 485–496.

EATON, W.W. AND WHITMORE, G.A. (1977). *Length of stay as a stochastic process: A general approach and application to hospitalization for schizophrenia. Journal of Mathematical Sociology*, **5**, 273–292.

© Springer Nature Switzerland AG 2022
W. Schwarz, *Random Walk and Diffusion Models*,
https://doi.org/10.1007/978-3-031-12100-5

EHRENFEST P. AND EHRENFEST, T. (1907). *Über zwei bekannte Einwände gegen das Boltzmannsche H-Theorem* [On two well-known objections against Boltzmann's H-Theorem]. *Physikalische Zeitschrift*, **8**, 311–313.

ERICH, R. AND PENNELL, M.L. (2015). *Ornstein-Uhlenbeck threshold regression models for time to event data with and without a cure fraction. Lifetime Data Analysis*, **21**, 1–19.

EWENS, W.J. (1977). *Urn models in genetics*. In: N.L. Johnson and S. Kotz, Urn Models and Their Application: An Approach to Modern Discrete Probability Theory (ch. 5.2). Wiley: New York.

FAMA, E.F. (1965). *Random Walks in Stock Market Prices. Financial Analysts Journal*, **21**, 55–59.

FICK, A. (1855). *Über Diffusion [On diffusion]. Poggendorfs Annalen der Physik und Chemie*, **94**, 59–86.

FISHER, R.A. (1922). *On the dominance ratio. Proceedings of the Royal Society of Edinburgh*, **42**, 321–341.

FÜRTH, R. (1920). *Die Brownsche Bewegung bei Berücksichtigung einer Persistenz der Bewegungsrichtung. Mit Anwendungen auf die Bewegung lebender Infusorien. [Brownian movement taking into account the persistence of movement. With applications to the movement of living infusoria]. Zeitschrift für Physik*, **2**, 244–256.

GABEL, A. AND REDNER, S. (2012). *Random walk picture of basketball scoring. Journal of Quantitative Analysis in Sports*, **8**, 1416.

GABRIEL, K.R. (1959). *The distribution of the number of successes in a sequence of dependent trials. Biometrika*, **46**, 454–460.

GOLD, J.I. AND SHADLEN, M.N. (2001). *Neural computations that underlie decisions about sensory stimuli. Trends in Cognitive Sciences*, **5**, 10–16.

GOLD, J.I. AND SHADLEN, M.N. (2007). *The neural basis of decision making. Annual Review of Neuroscience*, **30**, 535–574.

HANNEKEN, J.W. AND FRANCESCHETTI, D.R. (1998). *Exact distribution function for discrete time correlated random walks in one dimension. Journal of Chemical Physics*, **109**, 6533–6539.

HELLAND, E. AND RAVIV, Y. (2008). *The optimal jury size when jury deliberation follows a random walk. Public Choice*, **134**, 255–262.

HELMHOLTZ, H. VON (1878). *Die Thatsachen in der Wahrnehmung [The facts in perception]*. In: Vorträge und Reden (1896), vol. 2, 4th ed. (pp. 213–247). Braunschweig: Vieweg

KACELNIK, A., VASCONCELOS, M., MONTEIRO, T. AND AW, J. (2011). *Darwin's 'tug-of-war" vs. starlings' "horse-racing": how adaptations for sequential encounters drive simultaneous choice. Behavioral Ecology and Sociobiology*, **65**, 547–558.

KAREIVA, P.M. AND SHIGESADA, N. (1983). *Analyzing insect movement as a correlated random walk. Oecologia*, **56**, 234–238.

KOHLRAUSCH, K.W.F. AND SCHRÖDINGER, E. (1926). *Das Ehrenfestsche Modell der H-Kurve* [The Ehrenfest model of the H-curve]. *Physikalische Zeitschrift*, **27**, 306–313.

LANCASTER, T. (1972). *A stochastic model for the duration of a strike. Journal of the Royal Statistical Society, Series A (General)*, **135**, 257–271.

LEE, M.T. AND WHITMORE, G.A. (2006). *Threshold regression for survival analysis: Modeling event times by a stochastic process reaching a boundary. Statistical Science*, **21**, 501–513.

MARMA, V.J. AND DEUTSCH, K.W. (1973). *Survival in unfair conflict: Odds, resources, and random walk models. Behavioral Science*, **18**, 313–334.

MILLER, J.O. (1982). *Divided attention: Evidence for coactivation with redundant signals. Cognitive Psychology*, **14**, 247–279.

MILLER, J.O. (1986). *Timecourse of coactiavtion in bimodal divided attention tasks. Perception and Psychophysics*, **40**, 331–343.

O'CONNELL, R.G., SHADLEN, M.N., WONG-LIN, K. AND KELLY, S.P. (2018). *Bridging neural and computational viewpoints on perceptual decision-making. Trends in Neurosciences*, **41**, 838–852.

PALMER, J., HUK, A.C. AND SHADLEN, M.N. (2005). *The effect of stimulus strength on the speed and accuracy of a perceptual decision. Journal of Vision*, **5**, 376–404.

PASSINO, K.M. AND SEELEY, T.D. (2006). *Modeling and analysis of nest-site selection by honeybee swarms: the speed and accuracy trade-off. Behavioral Ecology and Sociobiology*, **59**, 427–442.

PELÉ, M. AND SUEUR, C. (2013). *Decision-making theories: linking the disparate research areas of individual and collective cognition. Animal Cognition*, **16**, 543–556.

POLSON, N.G. AND STERN, H.S. (2015). *The implied volatility of a sports game. Journal of Quantitative Analysis in Sports*, **11**, 145–153.

POTTIER, N. (1996). *Analytic study of the effect of persistence on a one-dimensional biased random walk. Physica A*, **230**, 563–576.

PRATT, S.C. (2005). *Quorum sensing by encounter rates in the ant Temnothorax albipennis. Behavioral Ecology*, **16**, 488–496.

PRZIBRAM, K. (1913). *Über die ungeordnete Bewegung niederer Tiere [On the random movement of lower animals]. Pflügers Archiv für Physiologie*, **153**, 401–405.

RATCLIFF, R. AND SMITH, P.L. (2004). *A comparison of sequential sampling models for two-choice reaction time. Psychological Review*, **111**, 333–367.

RATCLIFF, R. SMITH, P.L., BROWN, S.D., AND MCKOON, G. (2016). *Diffusion decision model: Current issues and history. Trends in Cognitive Sciences*, **20**, 260–281.

REIKE, D. AND SCHWARZ, W. (2016). *One model fits all: Explaining many aspects of number comparison within a single coherent model – A random walk account. Journal of Experimental Psychology: Learning, Memory and Cognition*, **42**, 1957–1971.

REIKE, D. AND SCHWARZ, W. (2019). *Aging effects on symbolic number comparison: No deceleration of numerical information retrieval but more conservative decision-making. Psychology and Aging*, **34**, 4–16.

SCHALL, J.D. (2001). *Neural basis of deciding, choosing and acting. Nature Reviews Neuroscience*, **2**, 33–42.

SCHALL, J.D., PURCELL, B.A., HEITZ, R.P., LOGAN, G.D. AND PALMERI, T.J. (2011). *Neural mechanisms of saccade target selection: gated accumulator model of the visual-motor cascade. European Journal of Neuroscience*, **33**, 1191–2002.

SCHRÖDINGER, E. (1915). *Zur Theorie der Fall- und Steigversuche an Teilchen mit Brownscher Bewegung [On the theory of experiments involving the fall and rise of particles undergoing Brownian movement]. Physikalische Zeitschrift*, **16**, 289–295.

SCHULTZ, C.B., PE'ER, B.G., DAMIANI, C., BROWN, L. AND CRONE, E.E. (2017). *Does movement behaviour predict population densities? A test with 25 butterfly species. Journal of Animal Ecology*, **86**, 384–393.

SCHWARZ, W. (1990). *Stochastic accumulation of information in discrete time: Comparing exact results and Wald–approximations. Journal of Mathematical Psychology*, **34**, 229–236.

SCHWARZ, W. (1991). *Variance results for random walk models of choice reaction time. British Journal of Mathematical and Statistical Psychology*, **44**, 251–264.

SCHWARZ, W. (1992). *The Wiener process between a reflecting and an absorbing barrier. Journal of Applied Probability*, **29**, 597–604.

SCHWARZ, W. (1993). *A diffusion model of early visual search: Theoretical analysis and experimental results. Psychological Research*, **55**, 200–207.

SCHWARZ, W. (1994). *Diffusion, superposition, and the redundant–targets effect. Journal of Mathematical Psychology*, **38**, 504–520.

SCHWARZ, W. (2001). *The Ex–Wald distribution as a descriptive model of response times. Behavior Research Methods, Instruments, and Computers*, **33**, 457–469.

SCHWARZ, W. (2002). *On the convolution of inverse Gaussian and exponential random variables. Communications in Statistics: Theory and Methods* , **31**, 2113–2121.

SCHWARZ, W. (2012). *Predicting the maximum lead from final scores in basketball: A diffusion model. Journal of Quantitative Analysis in Sports*, **8**, 1437.

SCHWARZ, W. AND MILLER, J. (2010). *Locking the Wiener process to its level–crossing time. Communications in Statistics: Theory and Methods*, **39**, 372–381.

SCHWARZ, W. AND STEIN, F. (1998). *On the temporal dynamics of digit comparison. Journal of Experimental Psychology: Learning, Memory, and Cognition*, **24**, 1275–1293.

SEELEY, T.D., VISSCHER, P.K. AND PASSINO K.M. (2006). *Group decision making in honey bee swarms: When 10000 bees go house hunting, how do they cooperatively choose their new nesting site? American Scientist,* **94**, 220–229.

SKELLAM, J.G. (1973). *The formulation and interpretation of mathematcal models of diffusionary processes in population biology.* In: The mathematical theory of the dynamics of biological populations. Eds. M.S. Bartlett and R.W. Hiorns. (pp. 63–85). London and New York: Academic Press.

SMITH, P.L. AND RATCLIFF, R. (2004). *Psychology and neurobiology of simple decisions. Trends in Neurosciences,* **27**, 161–168.

SMITH, A. AND STAM, A.C. (2004). *Bargaining and the nature of war. The Journal of Conflict Resolution,* **48**, 783–813.

SMOLUCHOWSKI, M. VON (1915). *Notiz über die Berechnung der Brownschen Molekularbewegung bei der Ehrenhaft-Millikan'schen Versuchsanordnung [Note on the calculation of Brownian molecular movement in the Ehrenhaft-Millikan experimental design]. Physikalische Zeitschrift,* **16**, 318–321.

STERN, H.S. (1994). *A Brownian motion model for the progress of sports scores. Journal of the American Statistical Association,* **89**, 1128–1134.

TAKACS, L. (1986). *Reflection principle.* In: Encyclopedia of Statistical Sciences, vol. 7 (pp. 670–673). Eds. S. Kotz and N. L. Johnson. John Wiley, New York, 1986,

TAYLOR, G.I. (1922). *Diffusion by continuous movements. Proceedings of the London Mathematical Society,* **20**, 196–212.

TSHISWAKA-KASHALALA, G. AND KOCH, S.F. (2017). *Contraceptive use and time to first birth. Journal of Demographic Economics,* **83**, 149–175.

TWEEDIE, M.C.K. (1945). *Inverse statistical variates. Nature,* **155**, 453.

WANG, M., BRENNAN, C.H., LACHLAN, R.F. AND CHITTKA, L. (2015). *Speed-accuracy trade-offs and individually consistent decision making by individuals and dyads of zebrafish in a colour discrimination task. Animal Behaviour,* **103**, 277–283.

WHITMORE, G.A., RAMSAY, T. AND AARON, S.D. (2012). *Recurrent first hitting times in Wiener diffusion under several observation schemes. Lifetime Data Analysis,* **18**, 157–176.

WHITMORE, G.A. AND NEUFELDT, A.H. (1970). *An application of statistical models in mental health research. Bulletin of Mathematical Biophysics,* **32**, 157–176.

WHITMORE, G.A. (1975). *The inverse Gaussian distribution as a model of hospital stay. Health Services Research,* **10**, 297–302.

WHITMORE, G.A. (1976). *Management applications of the inverse gaussian distribution. International Journal of Management Science,* **4**, 215–223.

WHITMORE, G.A. (1979). *An inverse gaussian model for labour turnover. Journal of the Royal Statistical Society, A,* **142**, 468–478.

WHITMORE, G.A. AND SESHADRI, V. (1987). *A heuristic derivation of the inverse Gaussian distribution. The American Statistician,* **41**, 280–281.

WOLF, M., KURVERS, R.H.J.M., WARD, A.J.M., KRAUSE S. AND KRAUSE, J. (2013). *Accurate decisions in an uncertain world: collective cognition increases true positives while decreasing false positives. Biological Sciences,* **280**, 1–9.

WRIGHT, S. (1931). *Evolution in Mendelian populations. Genetics,* **16**, 97–159.

YASUDA, N. (1975). *The random walk model of human migration. Theoretical Population Biology,* **7**, 156–167.

ZYLBERBERG, A., FETSCH, C.R. AND SHADLEN, M.N. (2016). *The influence of evidence volatility on choice, reaction time and confidence in a perceptual decision. eLife,* **5**, e17688.

Index

A

Absorbing barrier, 20, 37–41, 53, 79–91,
  96–111, 113, 114, 116, 118, 119,
  125, 136, 141, 144–165, 190, 195,
  197
Absorption probability in correlated random
  walk, 37–39, 41
Absorption probability in discrete random
  walk, 19–23
Absorption probability in general diffusion
  processes, 143, 150–151, 164
Absorption probability in Wiener process,
  97–98
Animal movement models, 1–2, 32, 173–176

B

Backward equation, 16–19, 60, 76–78, 85–87,
  115, 124, 125, 149
Backward process, 111–115
Batting average in baseball, 167–169
Brownian bridge, 118
Brownian motion, 1

C

Central limit theorem, 6, 15, 16, 59, 78, 99
Chapman-Kolmogorov equation, 127
Chi-square distribution, 69, 174
Coactivation models of information processing,
  188–190
Collective decision making, 4, 186, 187
Color discrimination in pigeons, random walk
  account of, 183–185
Conditional accuracy function (CAF), 196

Conditional maximum of Wiener process, 118,
  119, 178, 179
Conditional variance formula, 42, 132, 196
Conflict, bargaining and negotiated settlements,
  random walk model of, 171
Continuation value of contraception, 172
Correlated random walk, 32–42
Cumulant generating function (cgf), 116, 117

D

Darling and Siegert equations, 27, 109,
  136–139, 141–166
Difference equations, 44, 48, 57–60
Diffusion equation, 8, 10–12, 57–63, 65, 76,
  80, 122, 124
Discrimination and choice behavior in animals,
  182–185
Duration of strikes, 171

E

Ehrenfest model, 6, 43–46, 126, 130, 139, 199

F

Fick's laws, 4, 8–11, 60–63, 69, 74–76, 80, 122
First hitting model, 169–172
First-passage time distribution in a Wiener
  process, 65–67, 79–90, 100–109,
  133–136
Fisher-Wright model of random genetic drift,
  46–50, 126, 131–133, 139, 140, 147,
  151, 155, 156
Fixation of genes, 4

Printed in the United States
by Baker & Taylor Publisher Services